AF255511

J Ru's

DOUCHBAGGERY
FRAT BOY
FANTASTIC
FIGURE
WORKOUT
PROGRAM

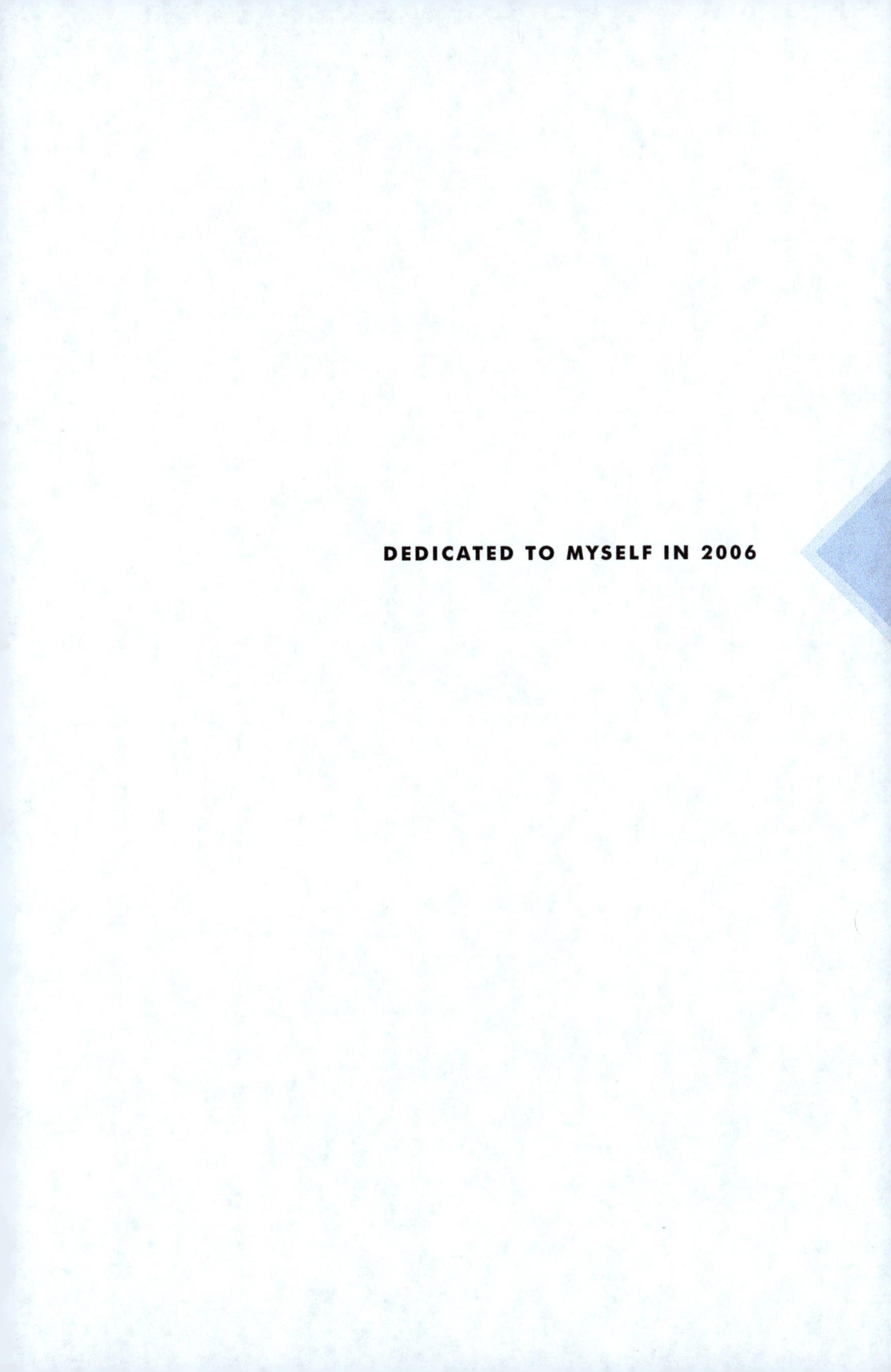

DEDICATED TO MYSELF IN 2006

CONTENTS

This book is about shifting perspectives.
I write this in hopes that at least one person, at some point in the future, will be able to cut down some of the time and research necessary to acquire and build the knowledge base of how to craft their very own perfect body. Bodies are imperfect places but striving for something better and higher brings us closer to the idea of perfection.

It took me ten years to research, test, consolidate and replicate my process, which I truly do feel that I was able to do. However I don't think that anyone should have to invest the same amount of time, that I did, into figuring it all out. I'm certainly not reinventing the wheel here by any means. All of the information is already out there. But that was always my very own problem: it's EVERYWHERE! The fitness world is overloaded with so much information that frankly it's hard to know where to start!

I don't want you to waste time. *Time*. That precious little thing we are all so delicately strapped by. Because once you achieve that perfect body that you've always wanted, the perfect body that the media have always led you to believe that you always needed, you'll realize, it was never your body that was the concern or problem in the first place, it was your perspective. And then you'll be able to move on from there.

But if you had told me not to be concerned about what my body looked like when it was shamefully, disgustingly, hopelessly, tumultuously, head-to-toe, covered in acne, I would have told you to eat dick and fuck yourself. Respectfully of course.

But before I get into the specifics, let me give you just a little more color...

HOW IT ALL BEGAN!

In my late teens, early twenties, like most kids, I developed acne. But unlike most kids, my acne was on a mission. My acne wanted to conquer, it wanted to colonize. It wanted to torment and harass. My acne succeeded in doing exactly that, all of it. No inch of my skin was safe from its war-like mission. There wasn't a dermatologist or Accutane prescription in the world that could help me. I truly tried every possible avenue.

For years to come, I could not look into the mirror without feeling a profound state of deep depression. It made me see myself as ugly, which was something I never ceased to stop telling myself either. Something I was reminded of every time I caught my reflection, every time someone snapped a photo, every time I opened my mouth.

I felt hopeless. I felt lost. I felt sad. I even felt depressed.

It became so intense that I even had suicidal thoughts roaming around my mind. All very gloomy!

Despite the shame, sadness, pain and even self-destruction that I honestly experienced, I didn't pull that trigger. Why? Because I didn't have the balls, and of course, I'm glad that I didn't... Deep down, I was hoping that these uncomfortable and overwhelming feelings would somehow pass. In the meantime I was, however, able to put my mind on a different track and shift my perspective. This is what I believe saved me from that depression cycle.

I told myself that...
If I could craft my body in such a way, that, I looked better than everyone else I knew, or could possibly come into contact with, based of course, on what the media had always portrayed for me as a "man's perfect body," then no one would notice how hideous I told myself I was. No one could make fun of me. No one would feel sorry for me. No one would be able to hurt me.

A perfect body would not change the vision I had of myself overnight and knit the confidence I needed in life, but I wouldn't have to hide anymore. I could go to the pool again. I could start dreaming the life I had always wanted... But I had to start with getting that perfect body. There simply wasn't another way... And so that's all that I focused on. Day in and day out. For years.

Eat. Train. Rest.
Eat. Train. Rest.
Eat. Train. Rest.

Consistency and dedication kept me focused. An approach you need to take too if you want to get the results you are after. As I worked hard, I quickly realized something I actually already knew. Achieving the body you've always desired is definitely not going to lead to your ultimate happiness. We all know this deep down, but it started a journey for me. As my body changed, my perspective changed and the meaning of a perfect body became so much more than what society tells you it is…

… still let's be honest, if you feel you must get there, then the following is a concise blueprint to achieving just that.

Tried. Tested. True.

J R
DOUCHE
FRAT
FANTASTI
WORKOUT

J'S
AGGERY
BOY
C FIGURE
PROGRAM

As I compiled all my research and my personal experience, I managed to create this 5-day cycle routine. Every detail counts and the exercise days are as important as the rest days. The fundamental idea is to not interrupt this workout cycle.

5-DAY CYCLE (TO BE REPEATED CONTINUOUSLY)

DAY 1	Lifting Dominant Day
DAY 2	Cardio Core Day
DAY 3	Lifting Dominant Day
DAY 4	Cardio Core Day
DAY 5	Rest Day

*A *Lifting Dominant Day* means that you should be focused on weight exercises only. A *Cardio Core Day* means your main goal is to complete a cardio routine. Super simple. Let's get started!

LIFTING DOMINANT DAY

Start with **15 to 20 minutes on the treadmill or stairmaster. It warms up your muscles and gets you going!**

Then choose 2 different Body Part Groupings. For example Chest and Bicep Groupings, or Back and Diverse Groupings. You want to work different parts of your body!

Each Body Part Grouping has 4 exercises. So get ready for 8 exercises in total!

Do 3 sets of each exercise.

And 15 Reps per set. If reps are not applicable, do the exercise for 1 minute. Set your timer!

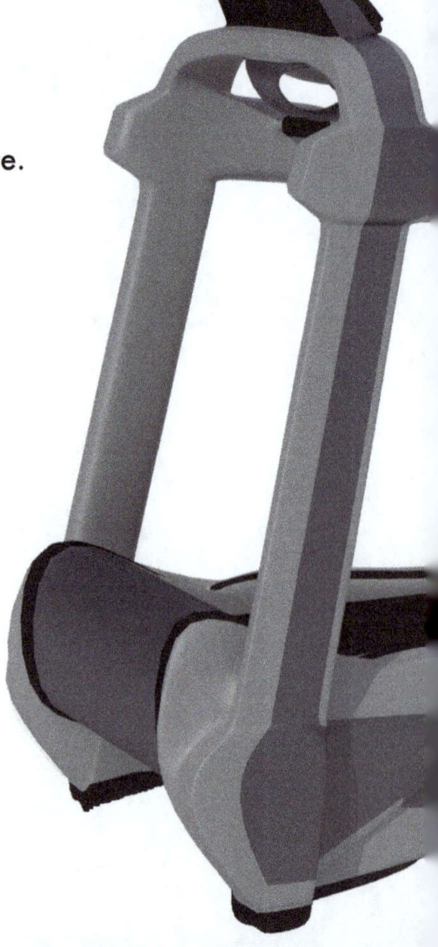

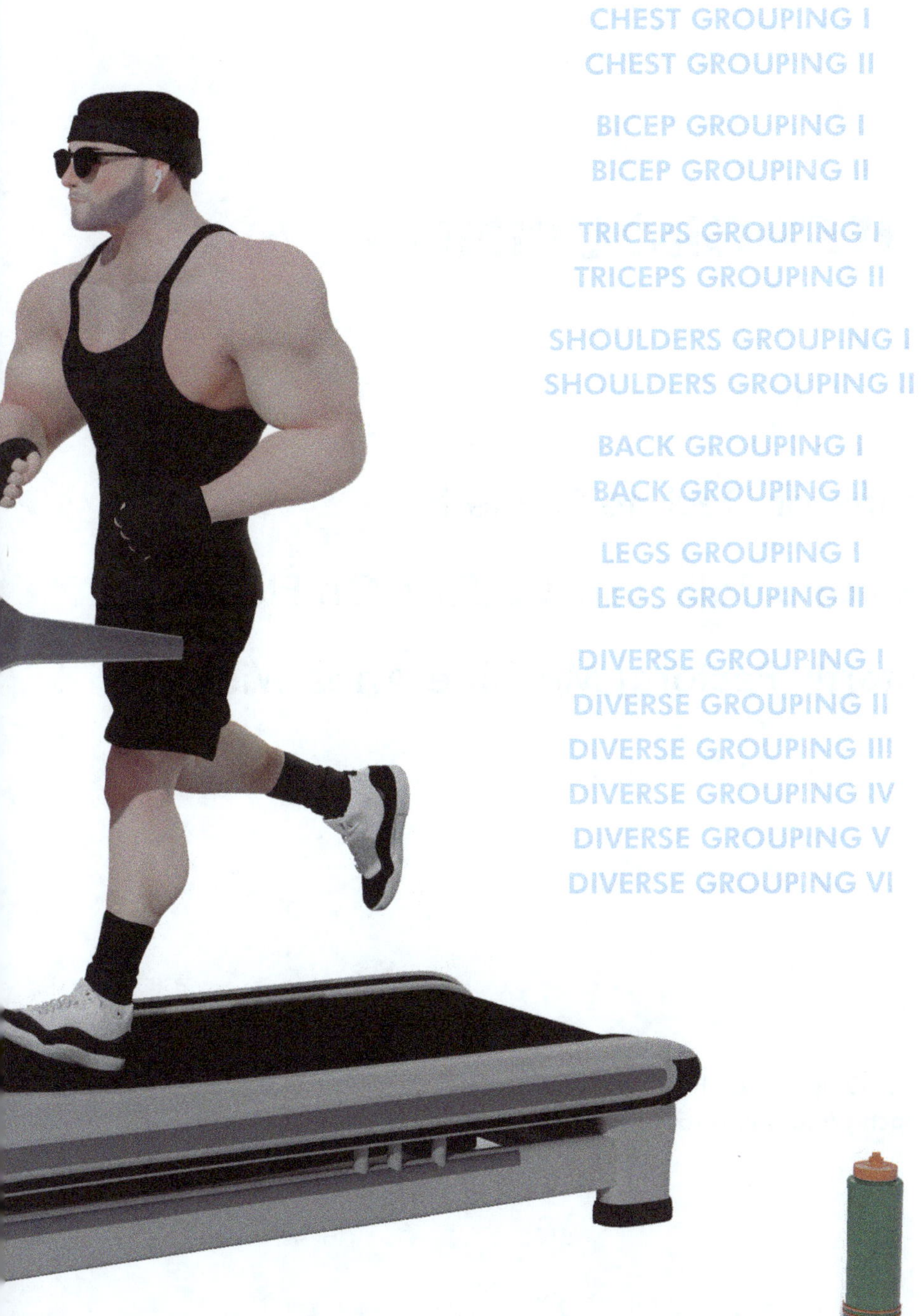

Here is a list of the Body Part Groupings for a Lifting Dominant Day:

CHEST GROUPING I

Barbell Bench Press

Incline or Decline Cable Fly

Medicine Ball Push-Up Pass On Floor

Butterfly Pectoral Machine Arms Wide

*NOTE: Only one of the four exercises
on each page is illustrated throughout.

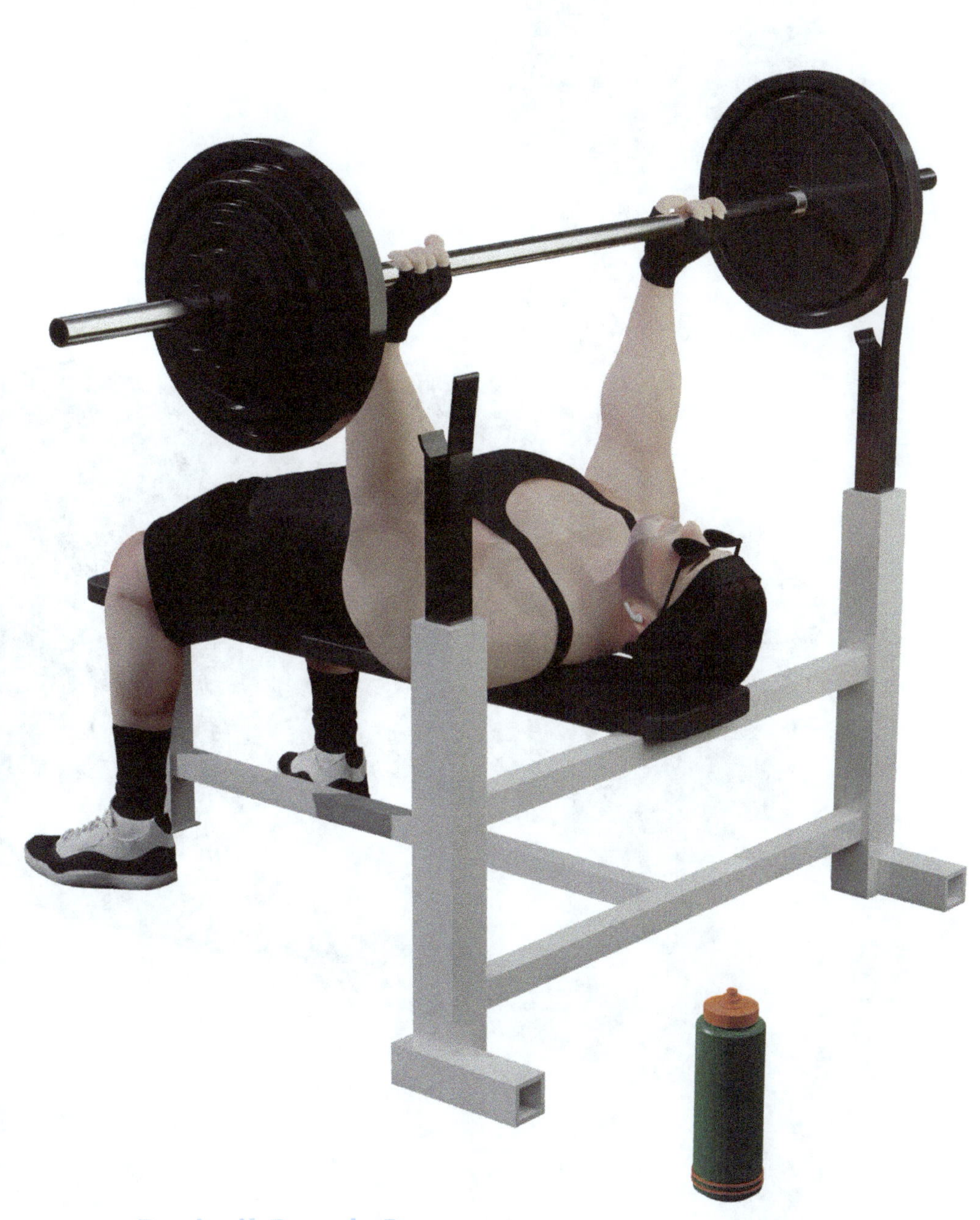
Barbell Bench Press

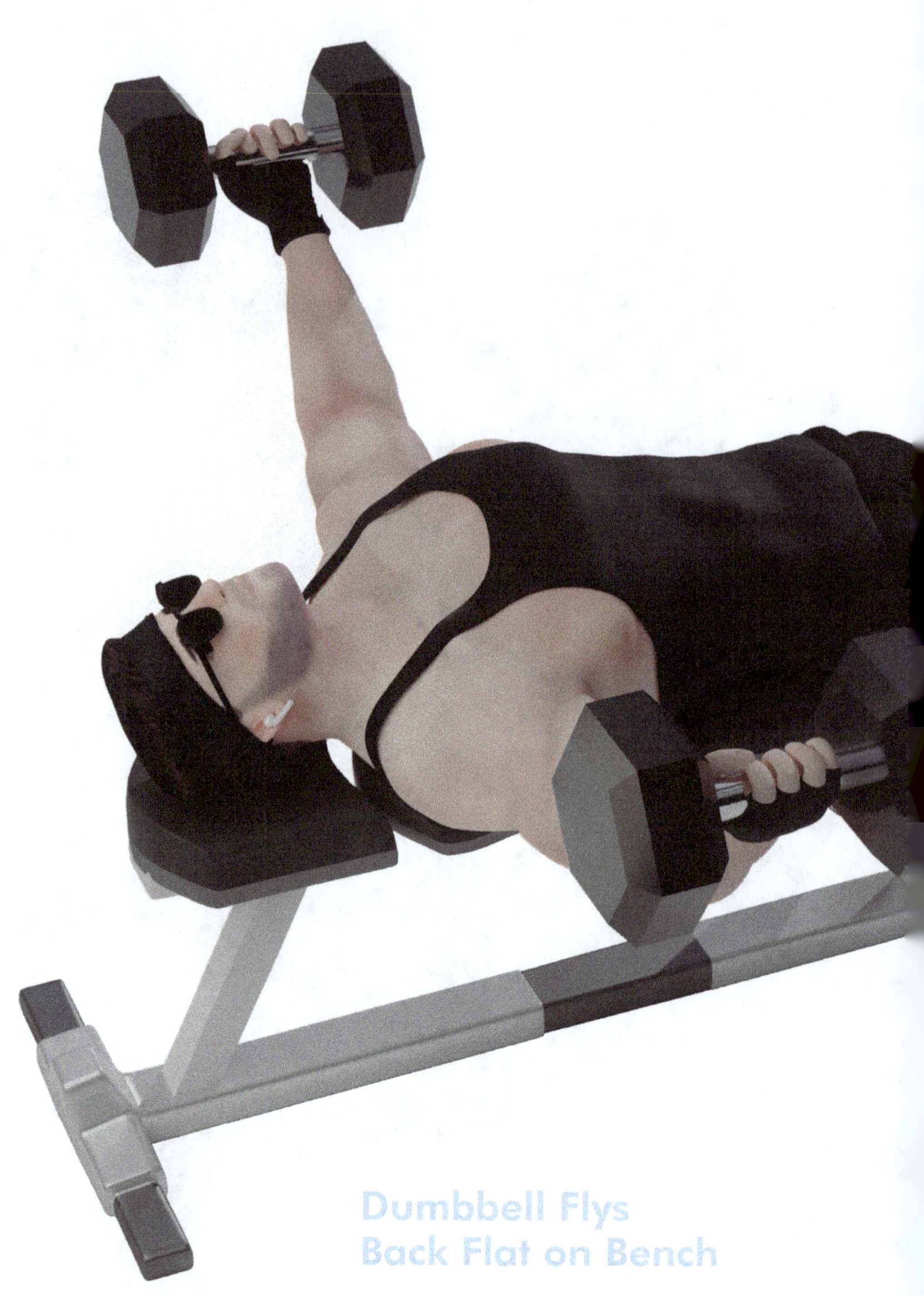

Dumbbell Flys
Back Flat on Bench

CHEST GROUPING II

Machine Bench Press

Dumbbell Flys Back
Flat on Bench

Decline Push-Up with
Weight on Back

Incline or Decline
Barbell Bench Press

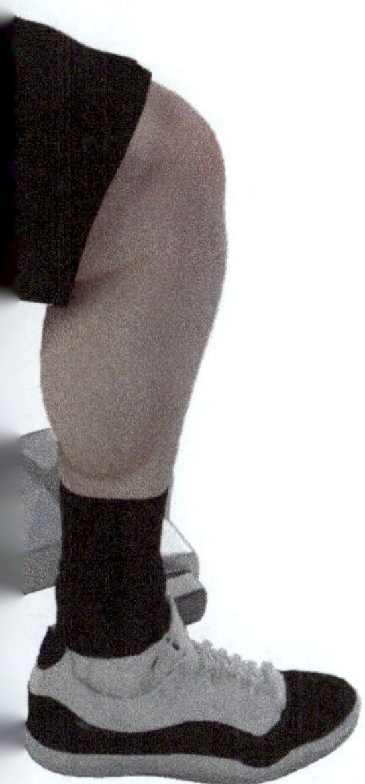

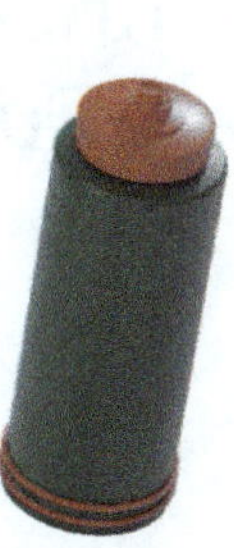

BICEP GROUPING I

Incline Dumbbell Hammer Curls

Internal or External Standing Dumbbell Curls

Standing Barbell Curls

Squatted (Elbow on Knee) Single-Arm Cable Concentration Curls

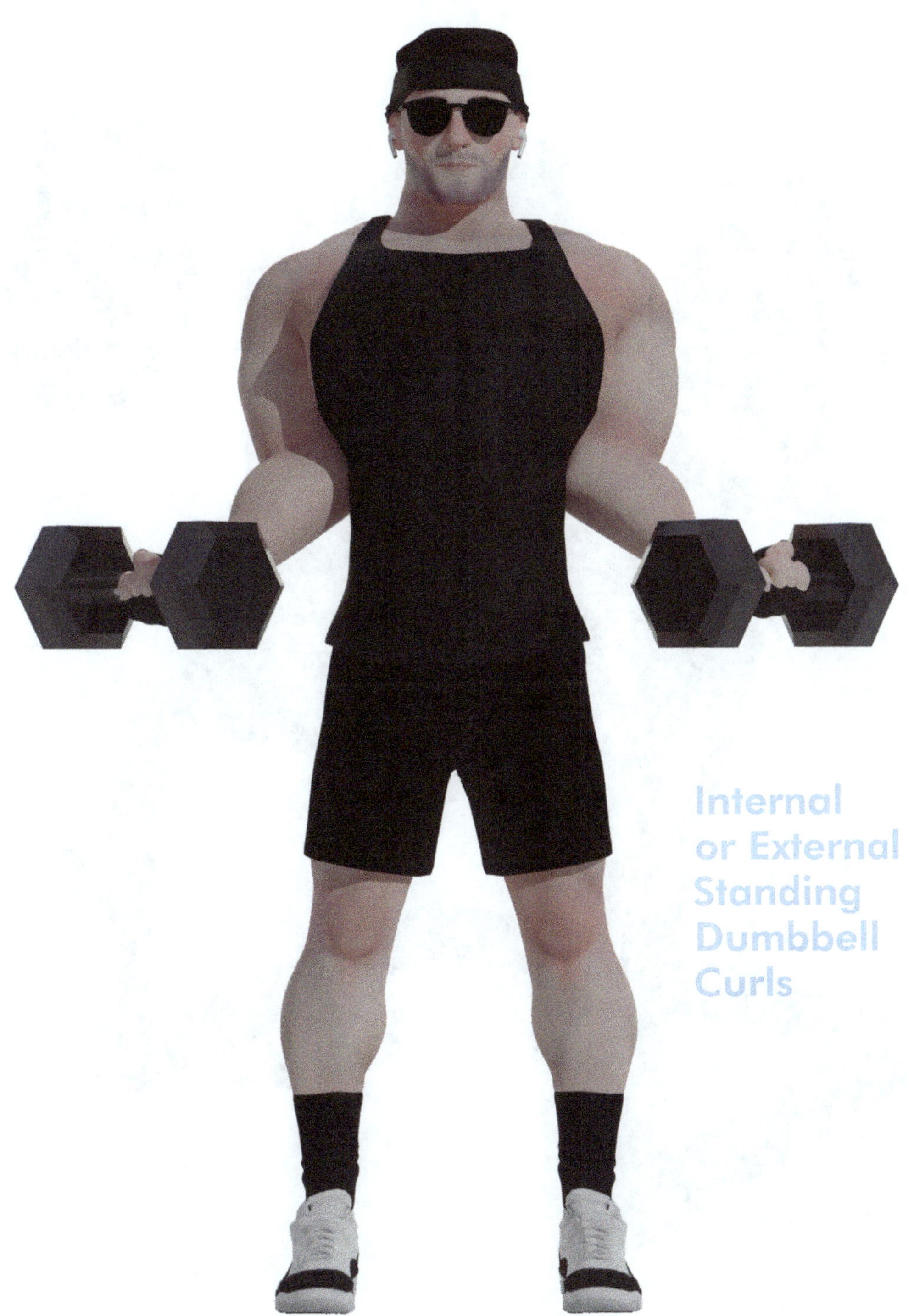

Internal
or External
Standing
Dumbbell
Curls

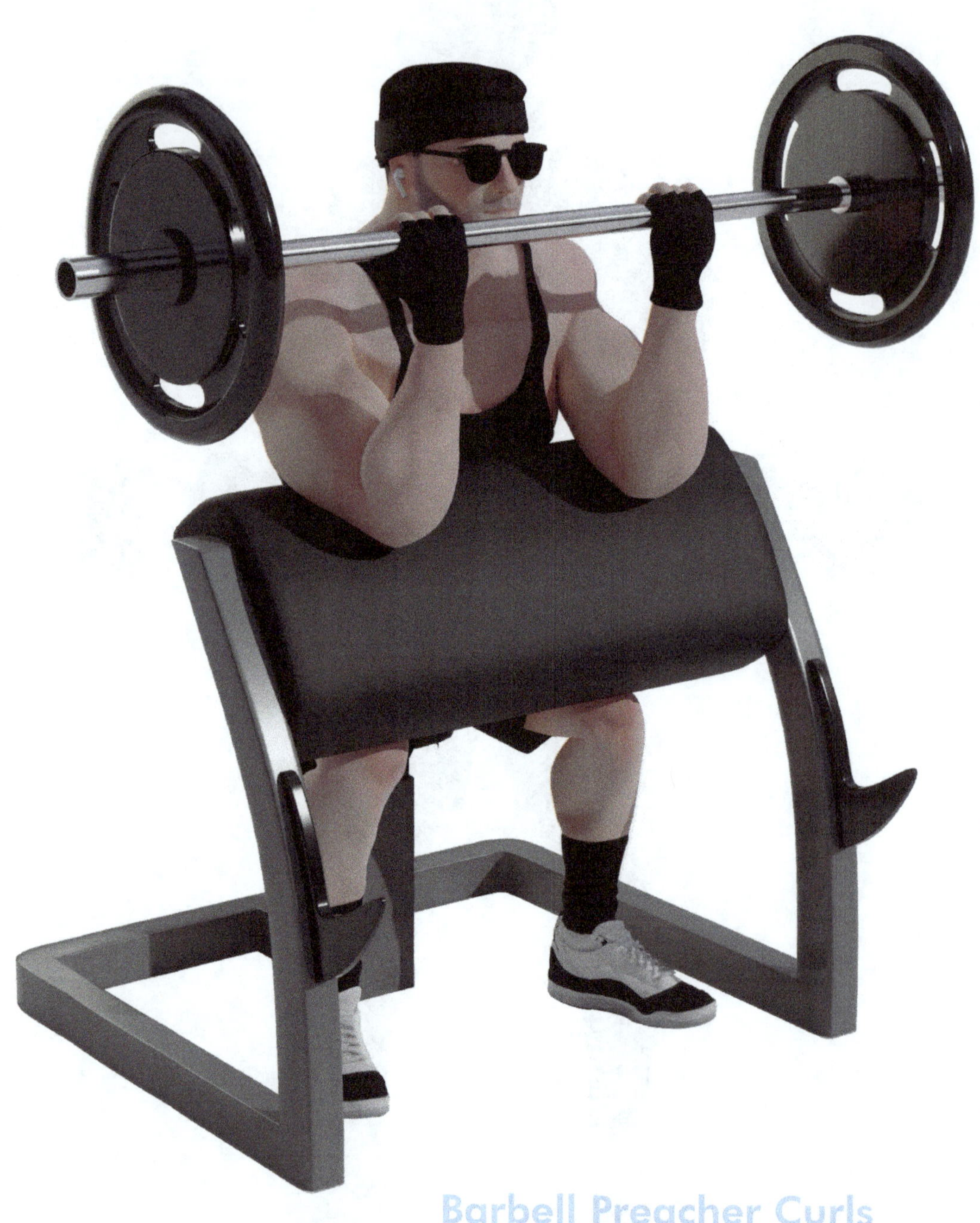

Barbell Preacher Curls

BICEP GROUPING II

Barbell Preacher Curls

Standing Overhead Cable Curl

Finish Position is Behind Head

Reverse Cable Curls

Start from Floor and Finish at Chest

Frontal Ferris Wheel Dumbbell Circle

TRICEPS GROUPING I

Rope Cable Push-Down & Out

Weighted Bench Dip with Feet on
Equal-Height Block

Seated Dumbbell
Overhead Triceps Press

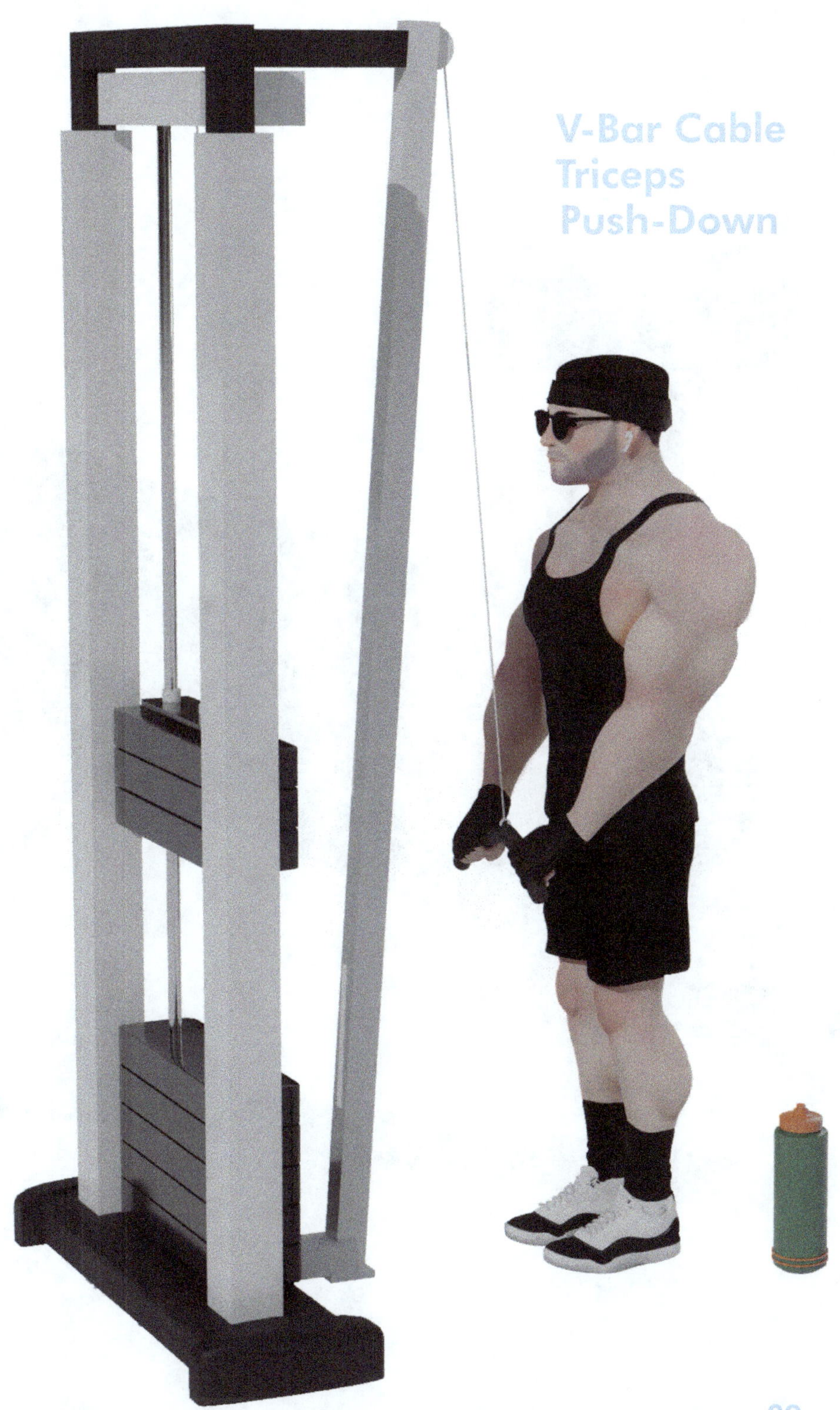

V-Bar Cable
Triceps
Push-Down

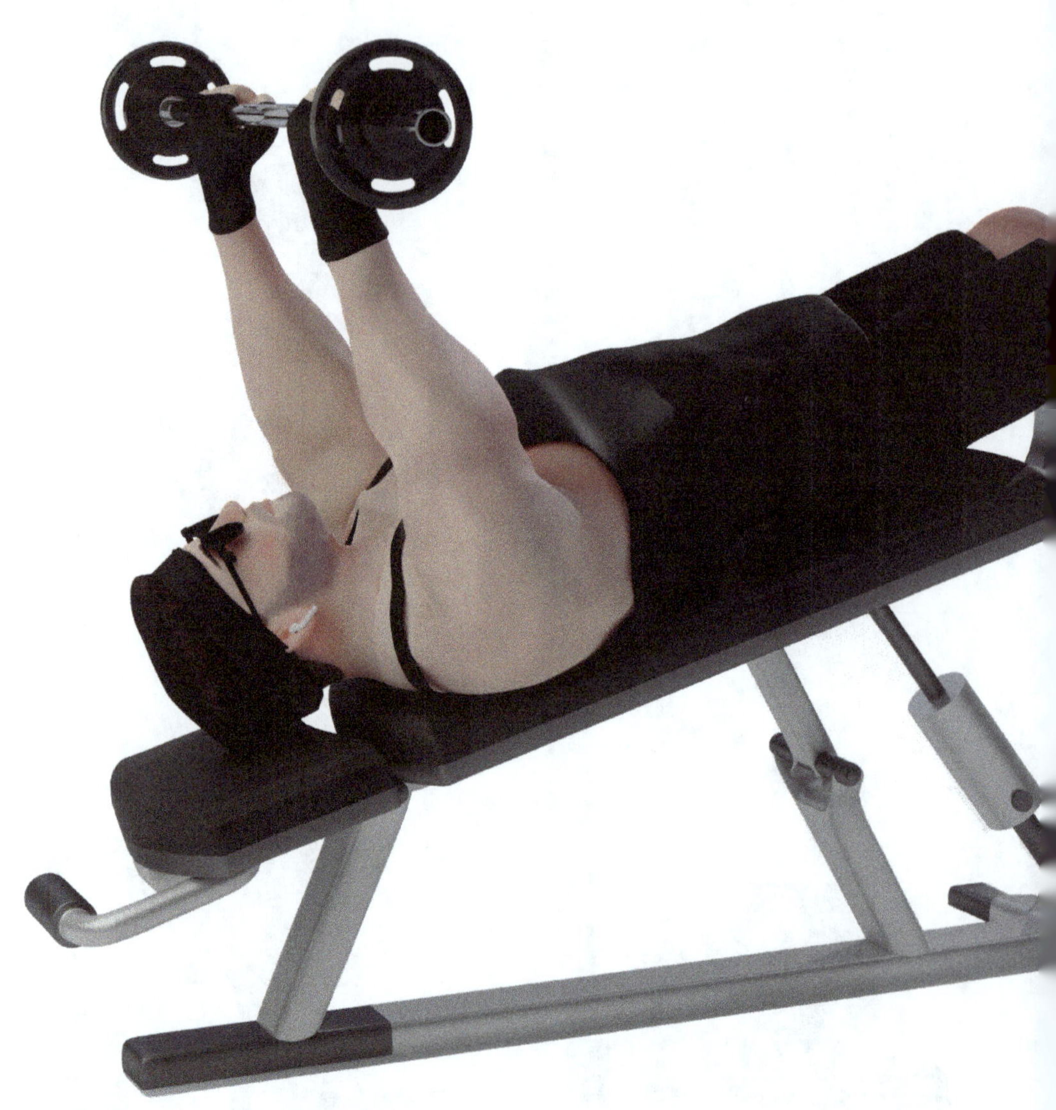

Decline Barbell Skull Crushers

TRICEPS GROUPING II

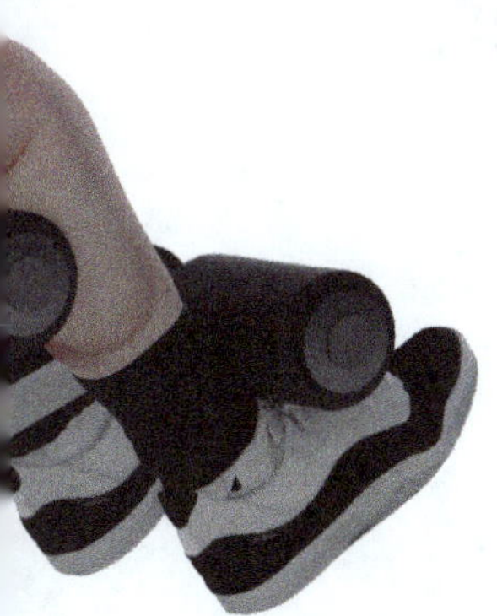

Cable Rope Overhead Triceps Extension

Dip Machine

One Arm Cable Push-Down

Decline Barbell Skull Crushers

Keep elbows locked in place

SHOULDERS GROUPING I

Seated Dumbbell Shoulder Press

**Standing Military Barbell
Overhead Press**

Front to Back then Back to Front

One Arm Cable Lateral Raise

Standing Upright Dumbbell Row

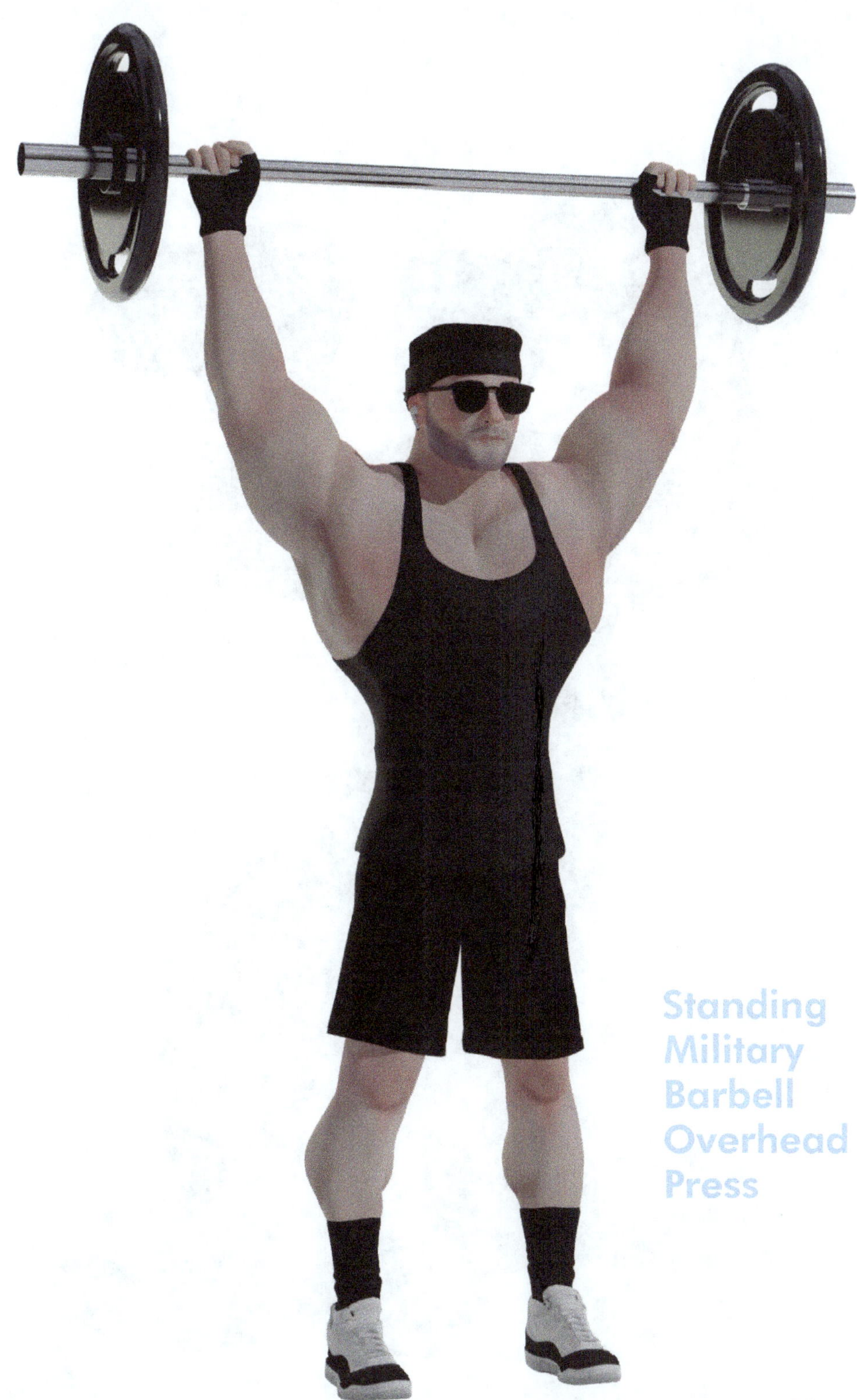

Standing
Military
Barbell
Overhead
Press

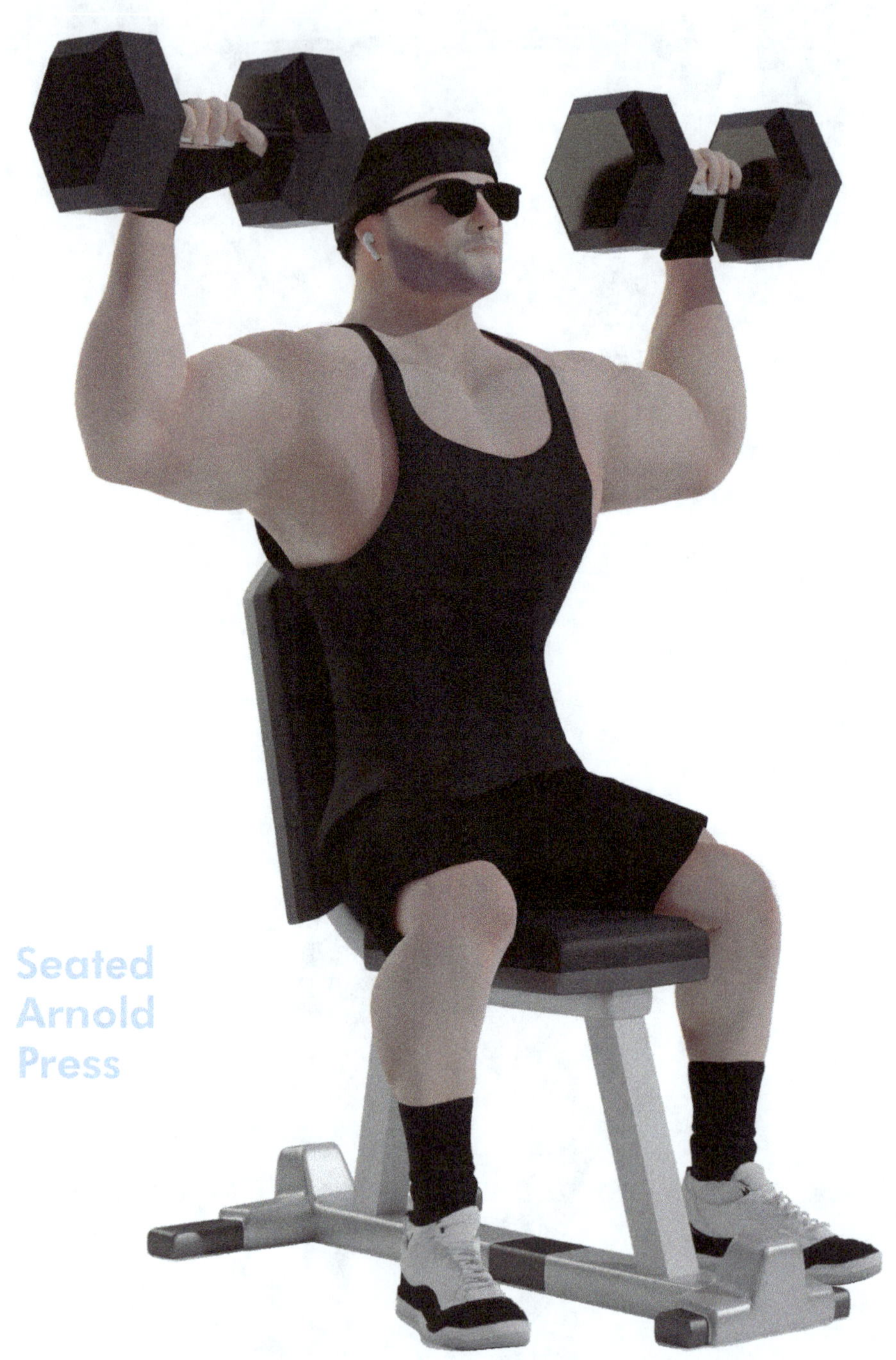

Seated
Arnold
Press

SHOULDERS GROUPING II

Single Arm Linear Jammers

Barbell Plate Car Drivers

Seated Arnold Press

Standing Military Barbell Overhead Press

Front to Back then Back to Front

BACK GROUPING I

Cable Wide-Grip Lat Pull-Down

Standing Cable or Sitting Machine Reverse Fly

One-Arm Dumbbell Row

1 Knee on Bench, 1 Leg Straight on Ground Back Flat

& Parallel to the Ground

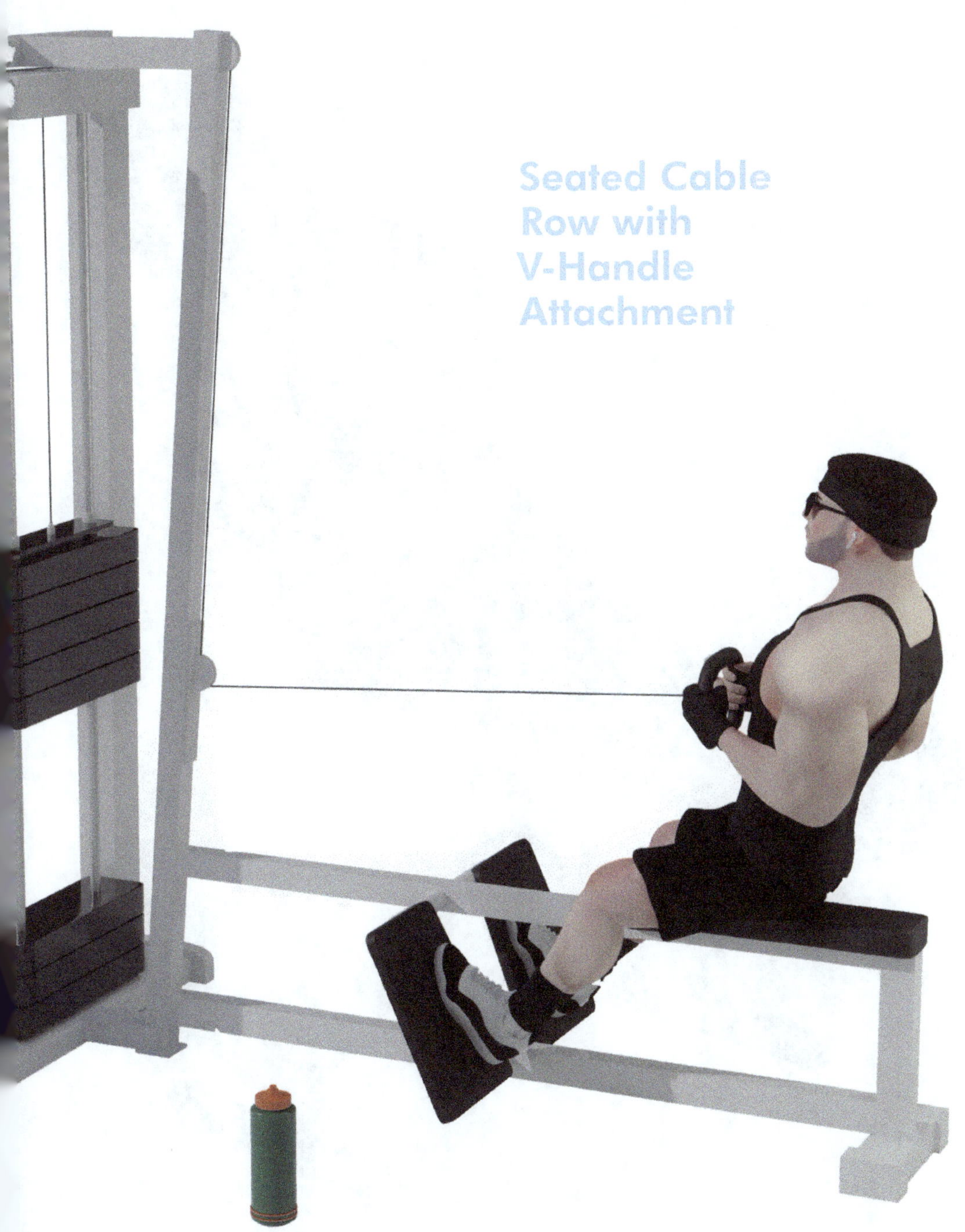
Seated Cable
Row with
V-Handle
Attachment

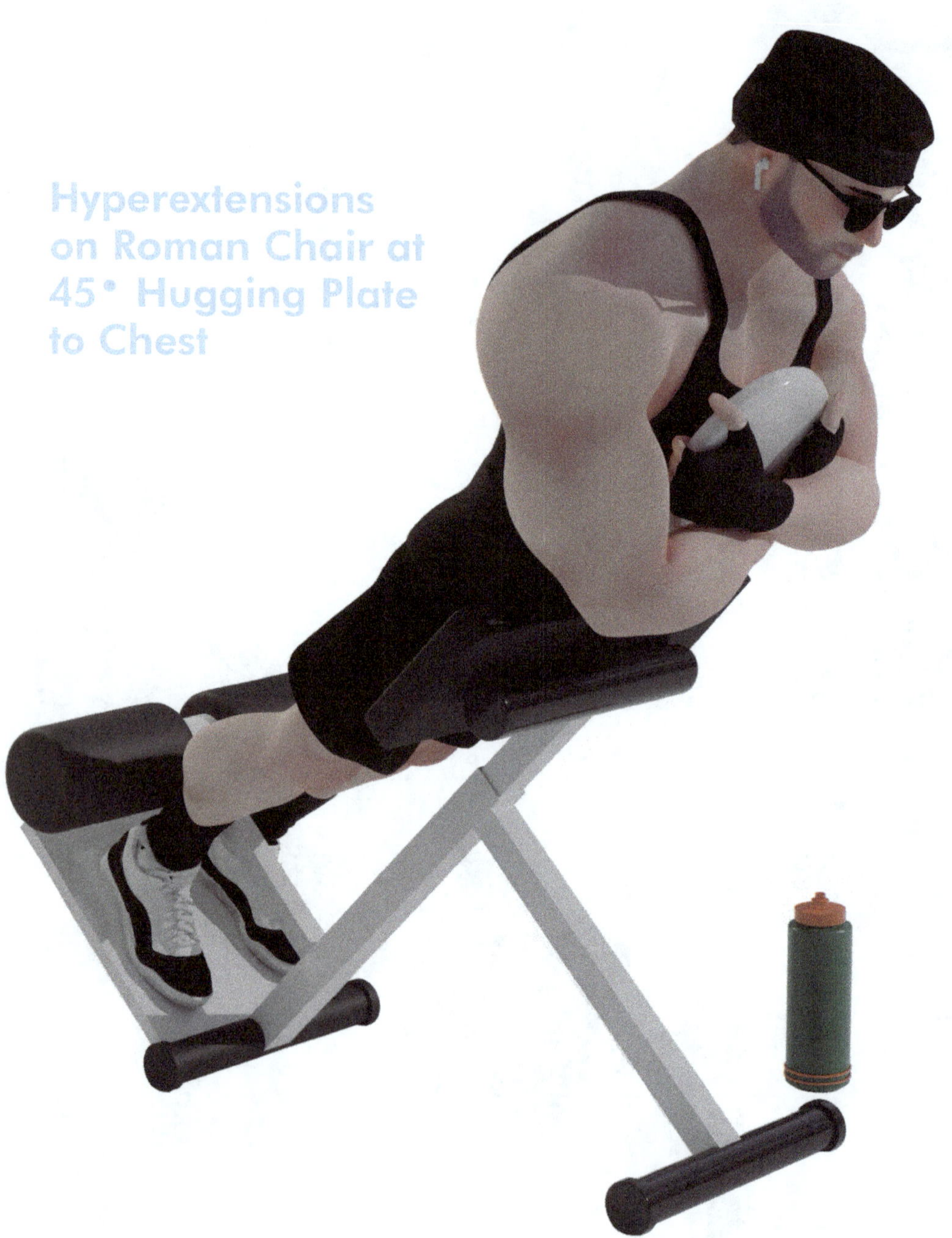

Hyperextensions
on Roman Chair at
45° Hugging Plate
to Chest

BACK GROUPING II

Machine T-Bar Rows

Hyperextensions on Roman Chair
at 45° Hugging Plate to Chest

Dumbbell Renegade Rows

Smith Machine Reverse Push-Up

LEGS GROUPING I

Leg Press

Walking Dumbbell Lunges

Standing Calf Raise

Side-To-Side Box Shuffle

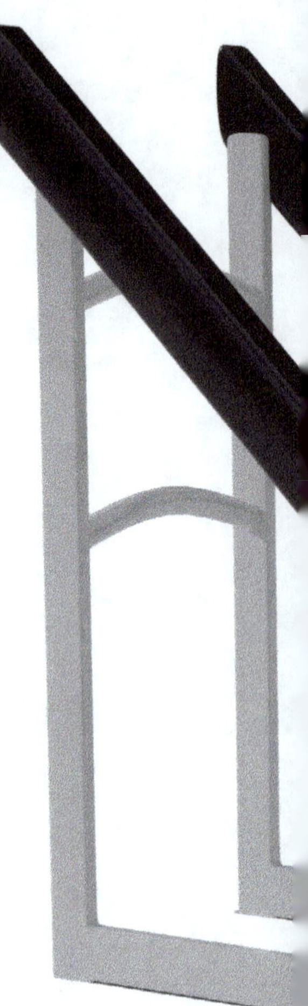

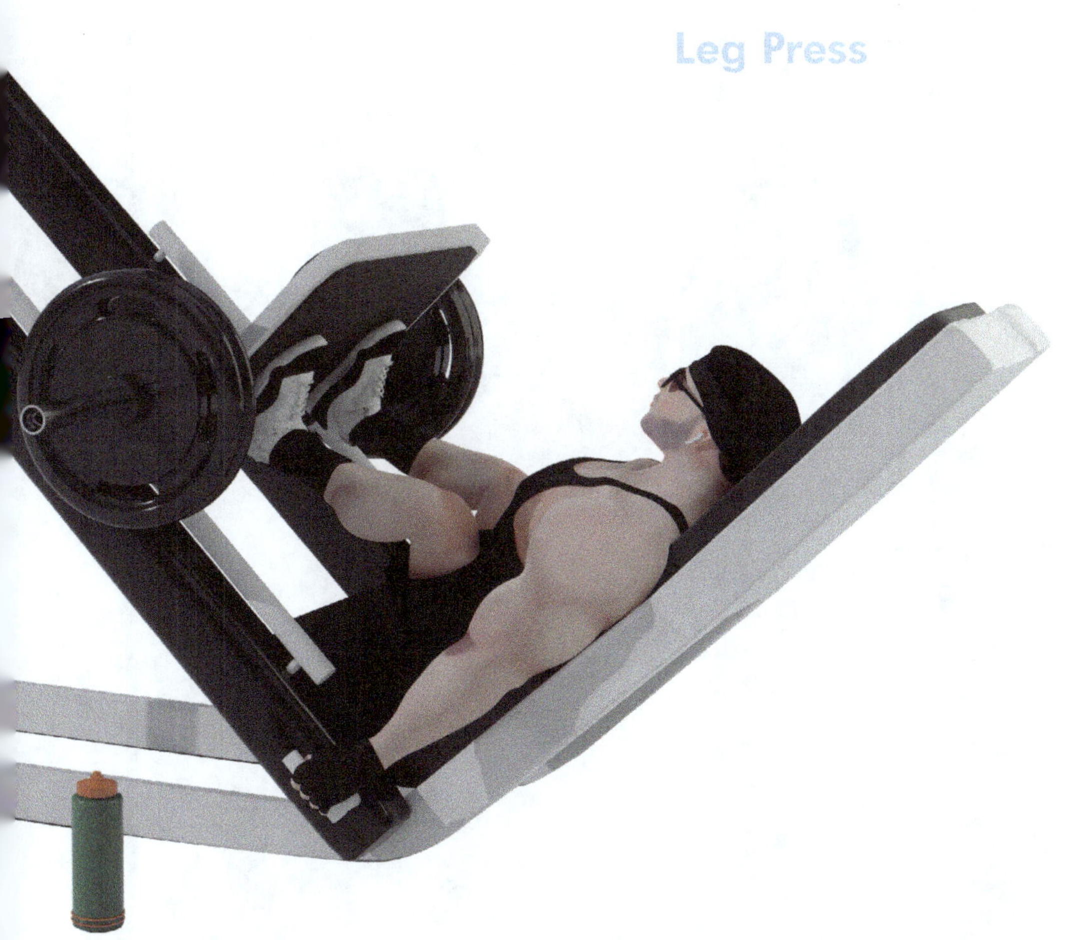

Leg Press

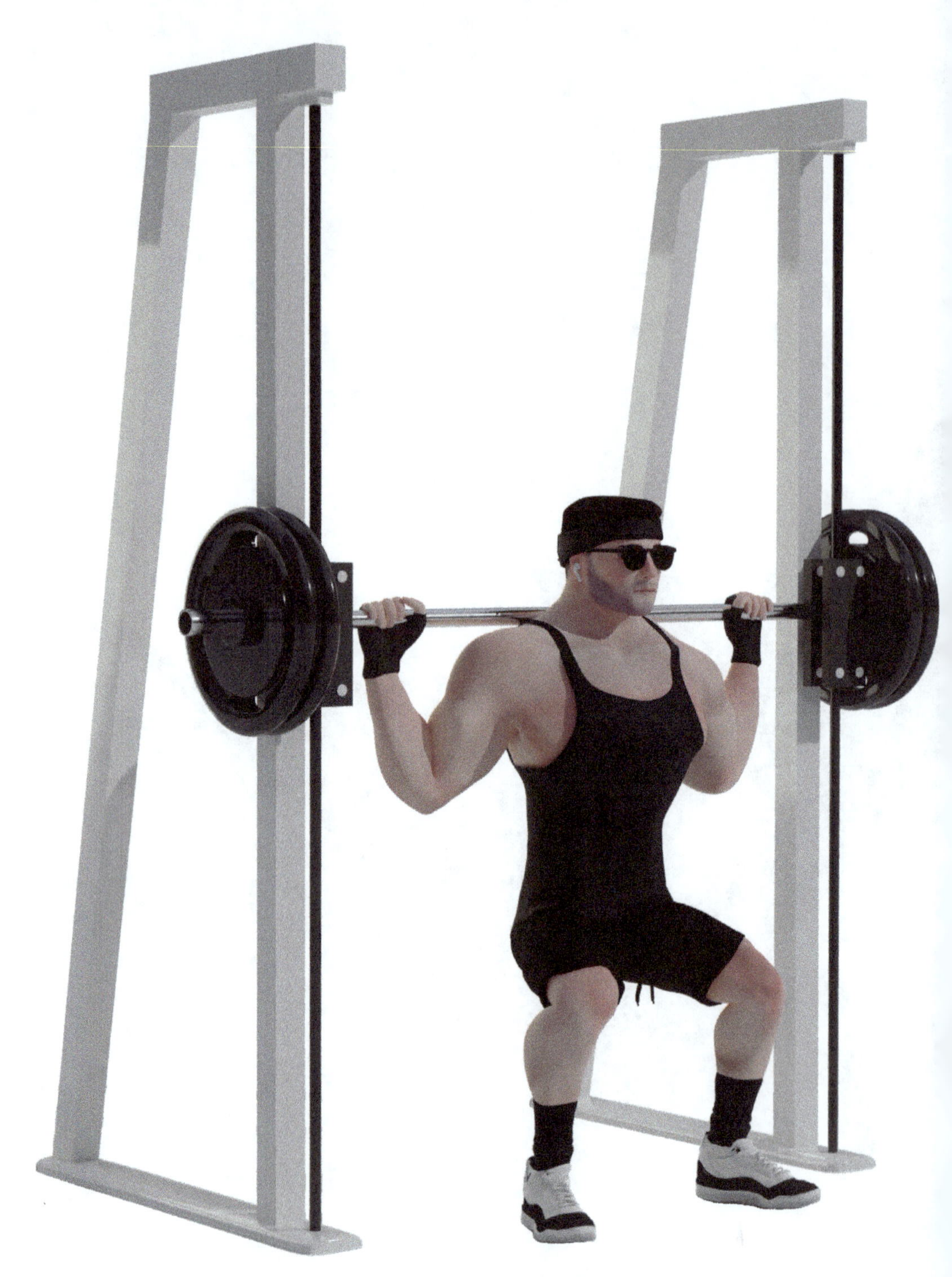

Smith Machine Squats

LEGS GROUPING II

Seated Leg Extension

Seated Hamstring Curl

Jump Box Burpees

Smith Machine Squats

DIVERSE GROUPING I

Rowing Machine

Dumbbell Farmer's Walk

Dips

Dumbbell Bicep Curl to
Shoulder Press

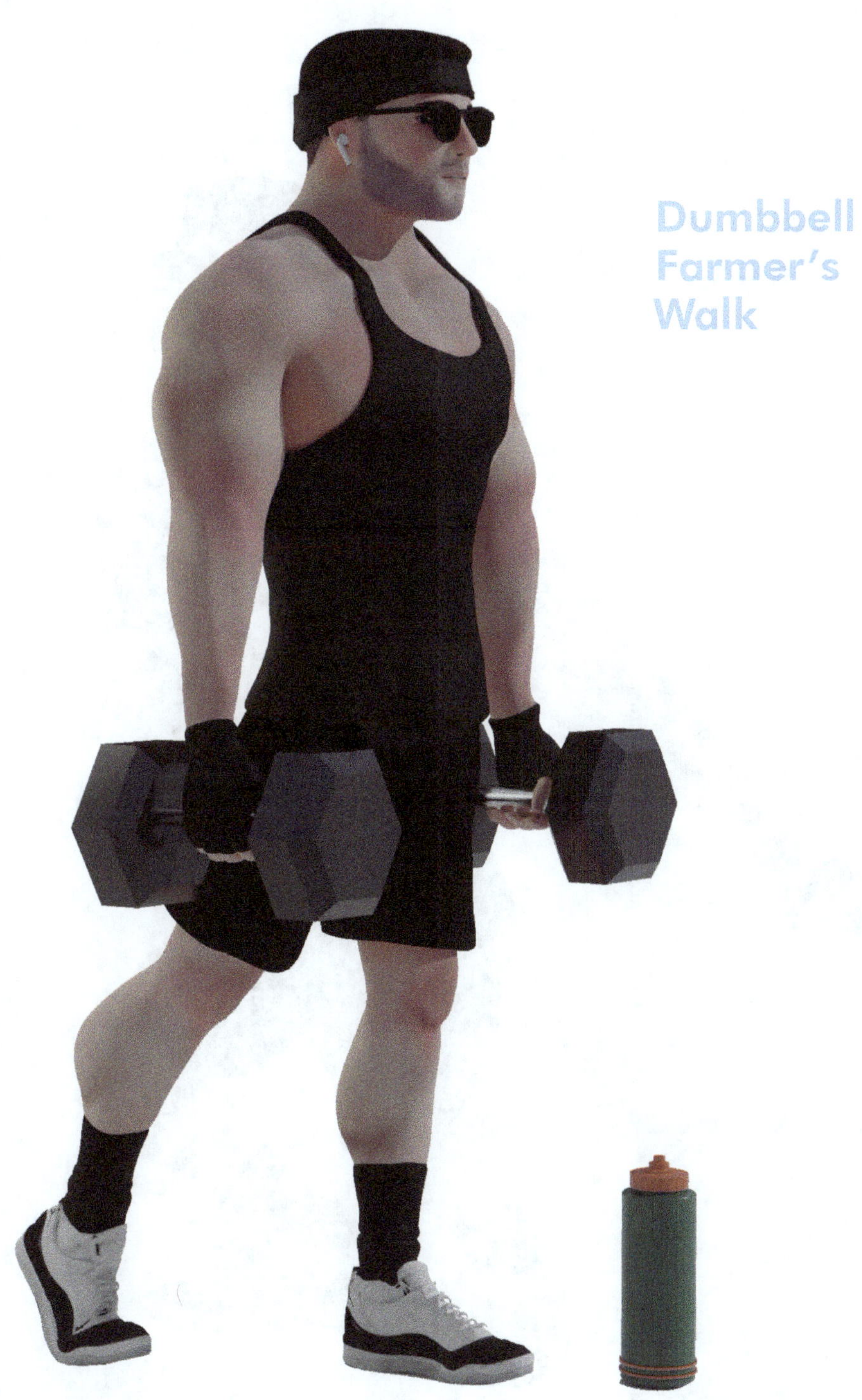

Dumbbell Farmer's Walk

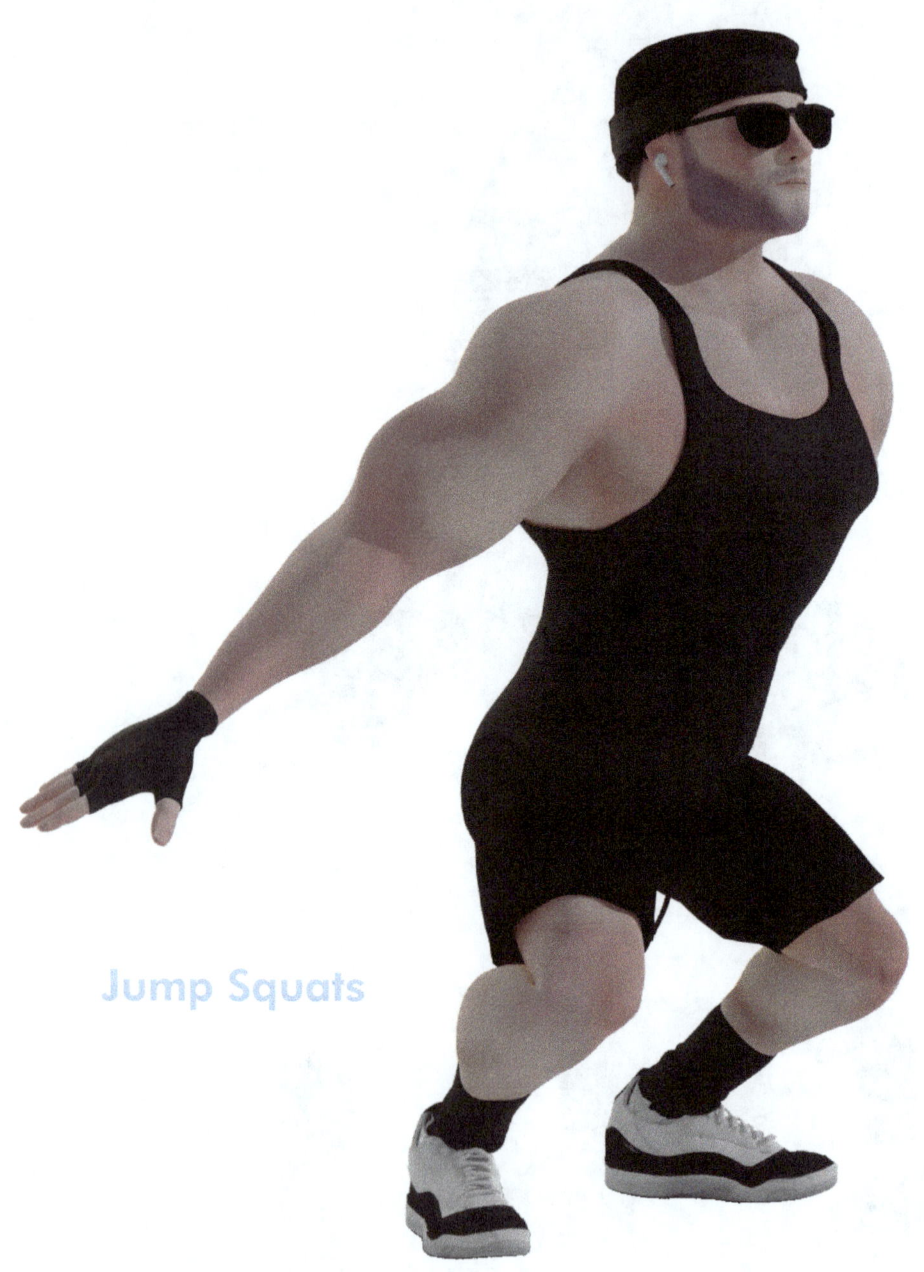

Jump Squats

DIVERSE GROUPING II

Hip Hinges

Jump Squats

Air Bike Crunches

Incline Push-Ups

DIVERSE GROUPING III

Elliptical

Jump Rope

Pull-Ups

Plank Shoulder Touches

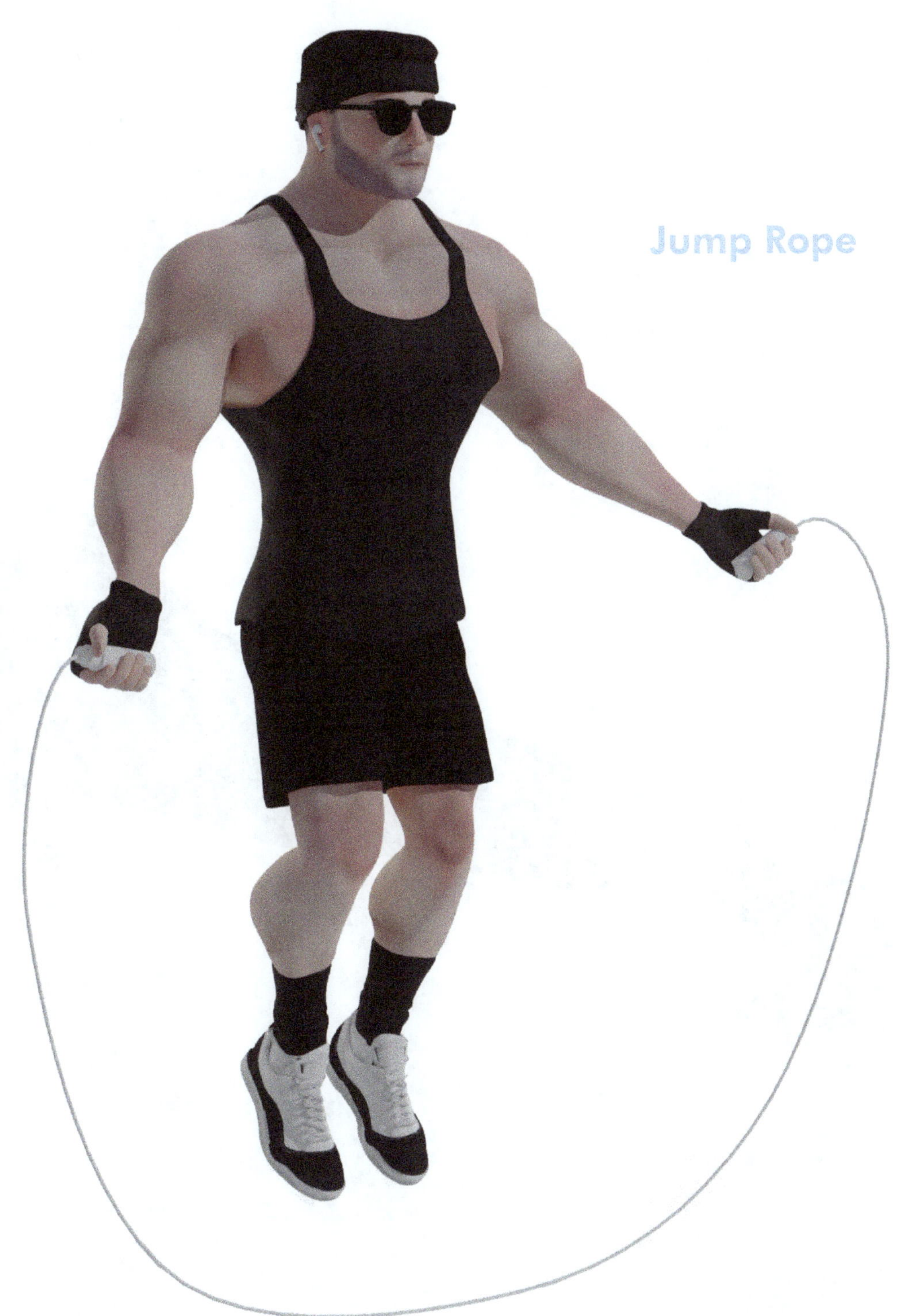

Jump Rope

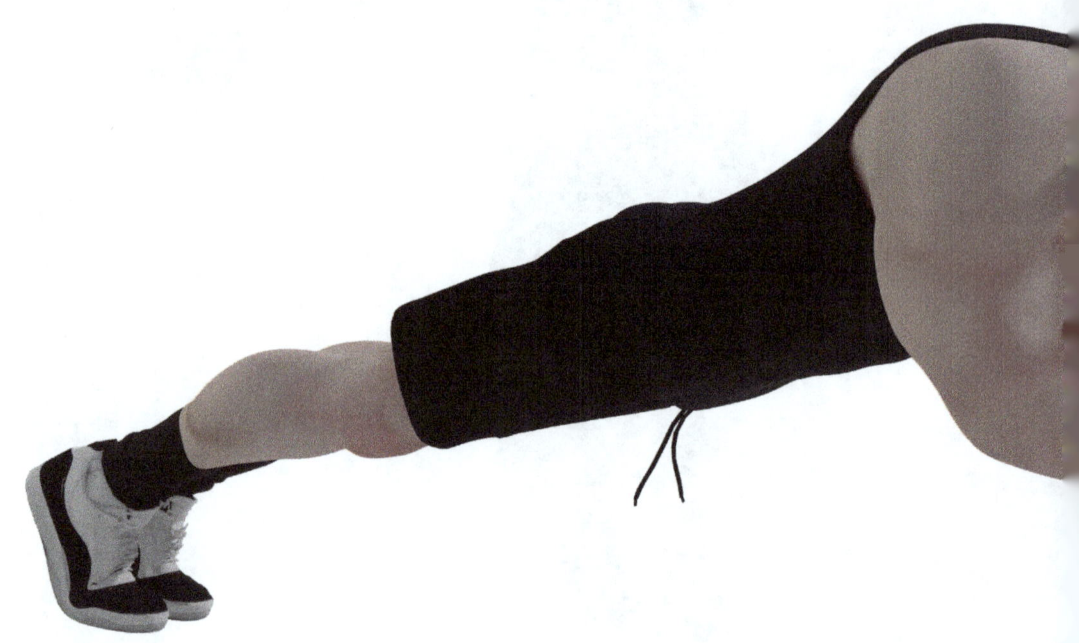

Clap Push-Ups

DIVERSE GROUPING IV

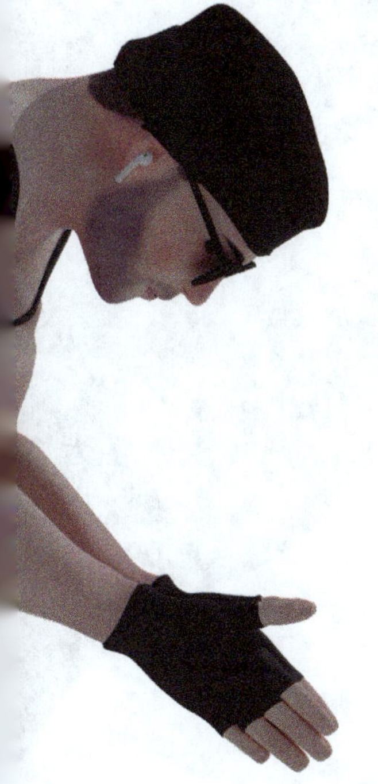

Clap Push-Ups

Smith Machine Shrug

Front & Back

Barbell Squat

Kettlebell 2-Arm High Pull

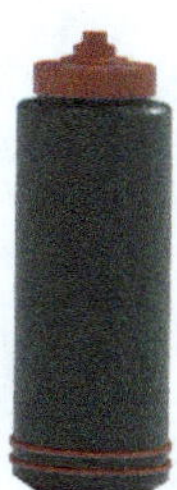

DIVERSE GROUPING V

Triangle Push-Ups

High Knees

Jumping Jacks

Sit-Ups

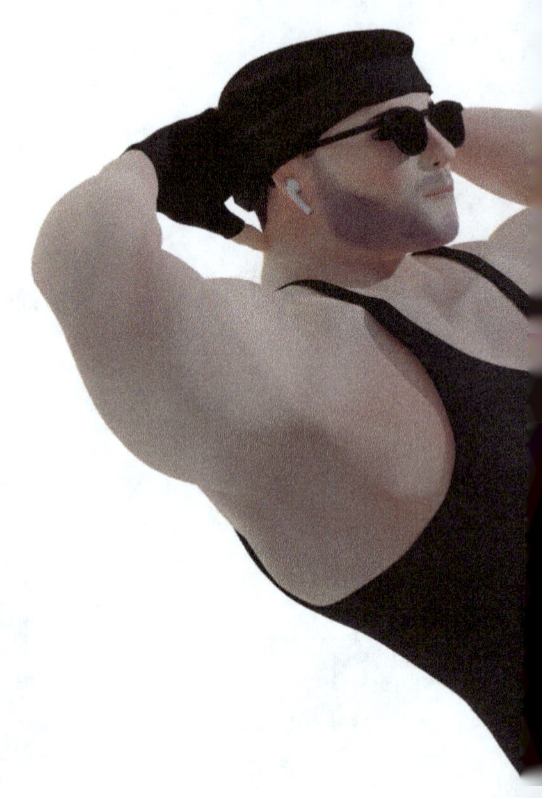

Sit-Ups

Bicycles

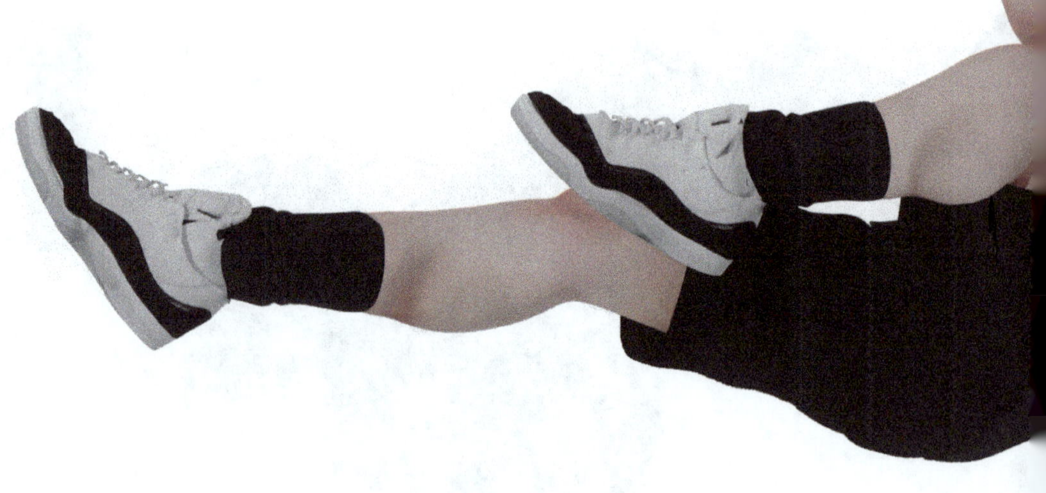

DIVERSE GROUPING VI

Bicycles

Sumo Squats

Heavy Dumbbell Trap Shrug

Light Dumbbell In-Place
Arm Sprinting Hammer Curls

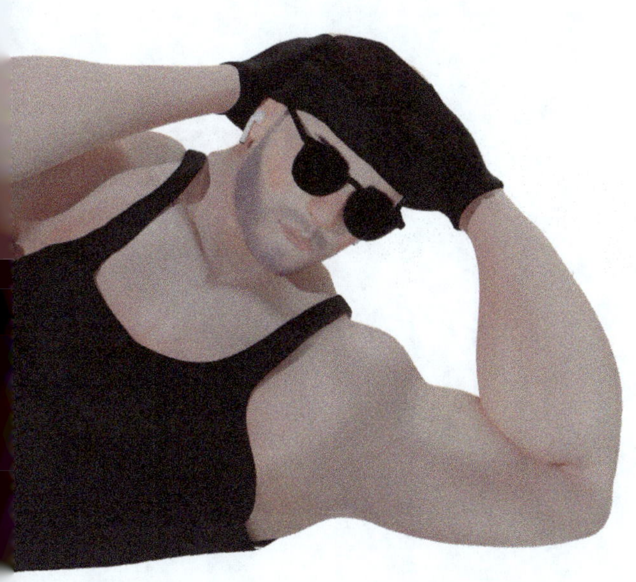

NO-NOS

Do not repeat the same Grouping Type until you have gone through all the different Groupings.

So if on Monday, you picked Chest and Shoulders, do not choose Chest and Shoulders until you have cycled through Biceps, Triceps, Back and Legs!

CARDIO CORE DAY

Choose 1 Cardio Set to do for 30 minutes.
Then choose 1 Core Grouping.
Each Grouping has 4 exercises.
1 Minute Per Set.

Here are the Cardio Sets:

CARDIO SETS

Treadmill Run

Stairmaster

Hill Sprints

Rowing Machine

      1 minute On, 1 minute Off

Jump Rope

      1 minute On, 1 minute Off

Here is a list of the different Core Groupings:

CORE GROUPING I
CORE GROUPING II
CORE GROUPING III
CORE GROUPING IV
CORE GROUPING V
CORE GROUPING VI

CORE GROUPING I

Landmine 180 Twists

Planks

Kneeling Cable Crunch with Alternating Oblique Twists

Barbell Rollout

Knees Elevated on Bench

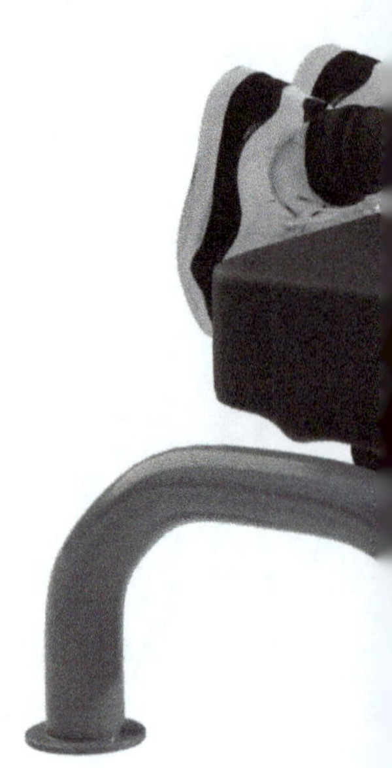

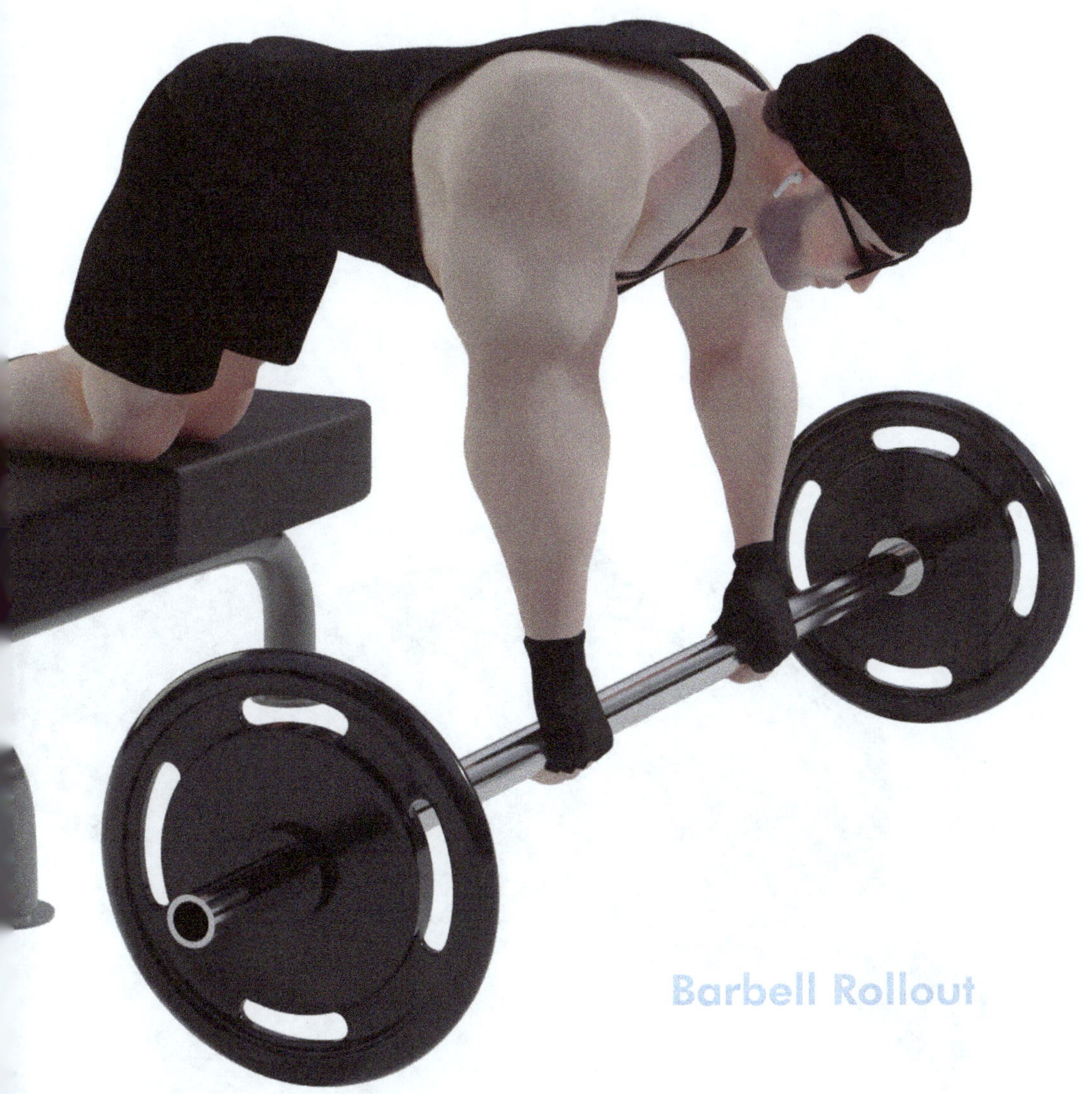

Barbell Rollout

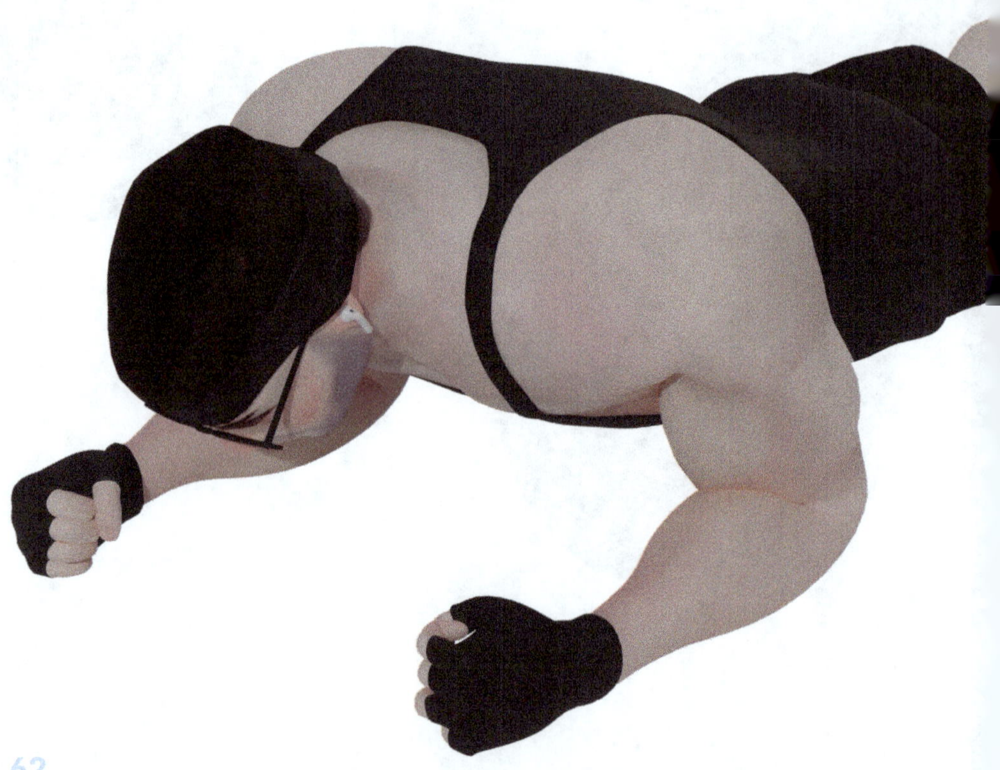

Weighted Planks

CORE GROUPING II

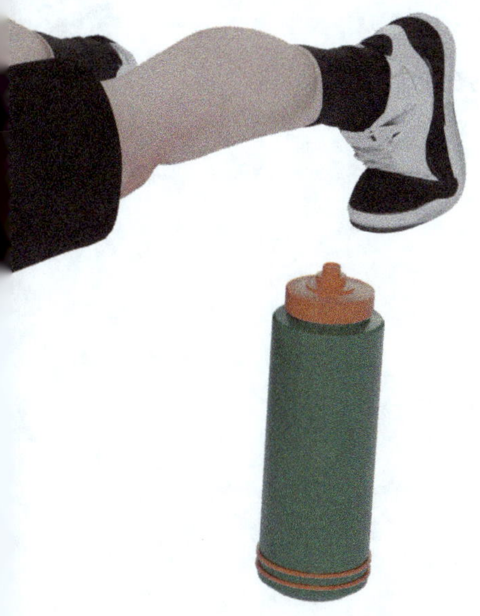

CORE GROUPING III

Decline Sit-Ups

Decline Bench Medicine Ball
Opposite Side Twist Throw (To Person)

Hanging Oblique Leg Raise

Standing Plate Twist

Keep Plate at Hip Level

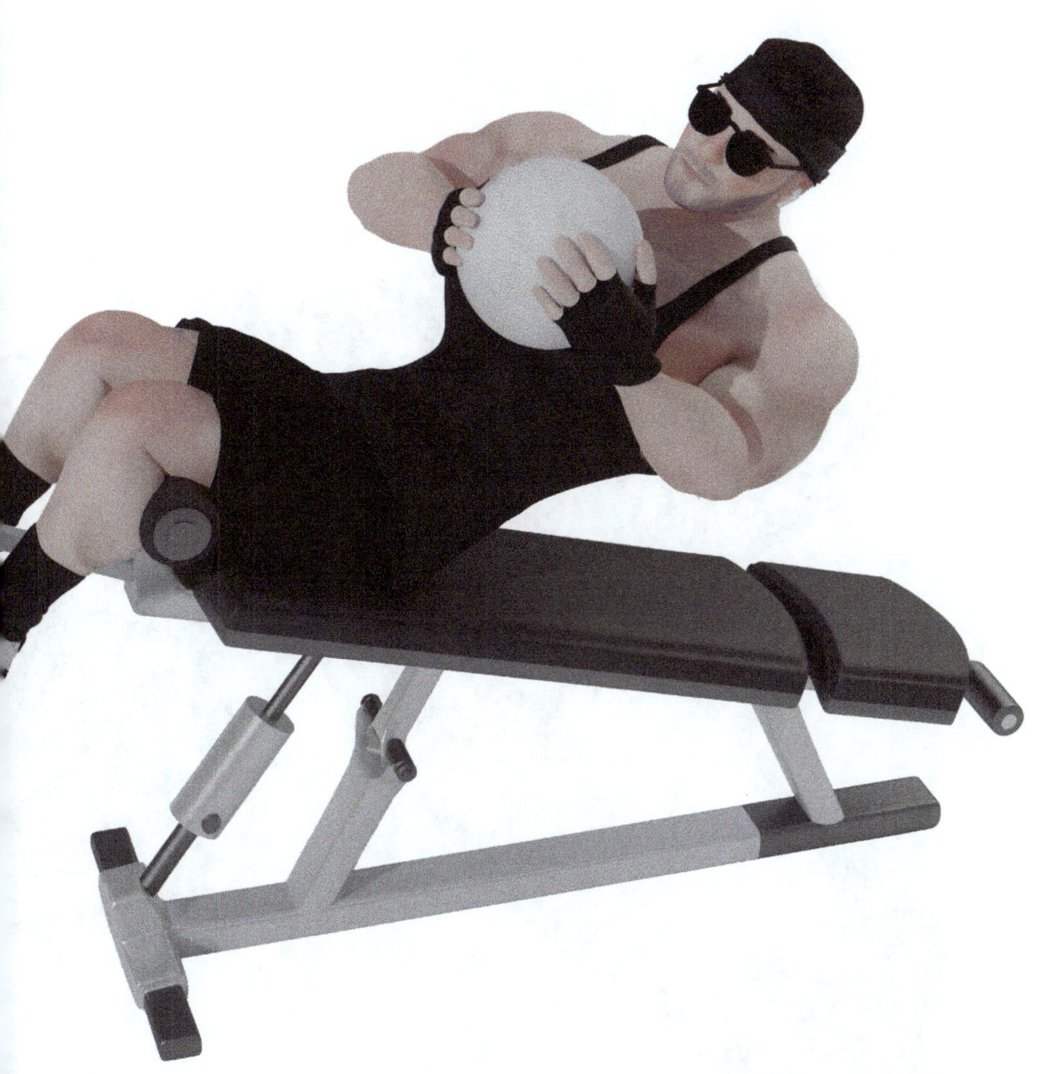

Decline Bench Medicine
Ball Opposite Side
Twist Throw (To Person)

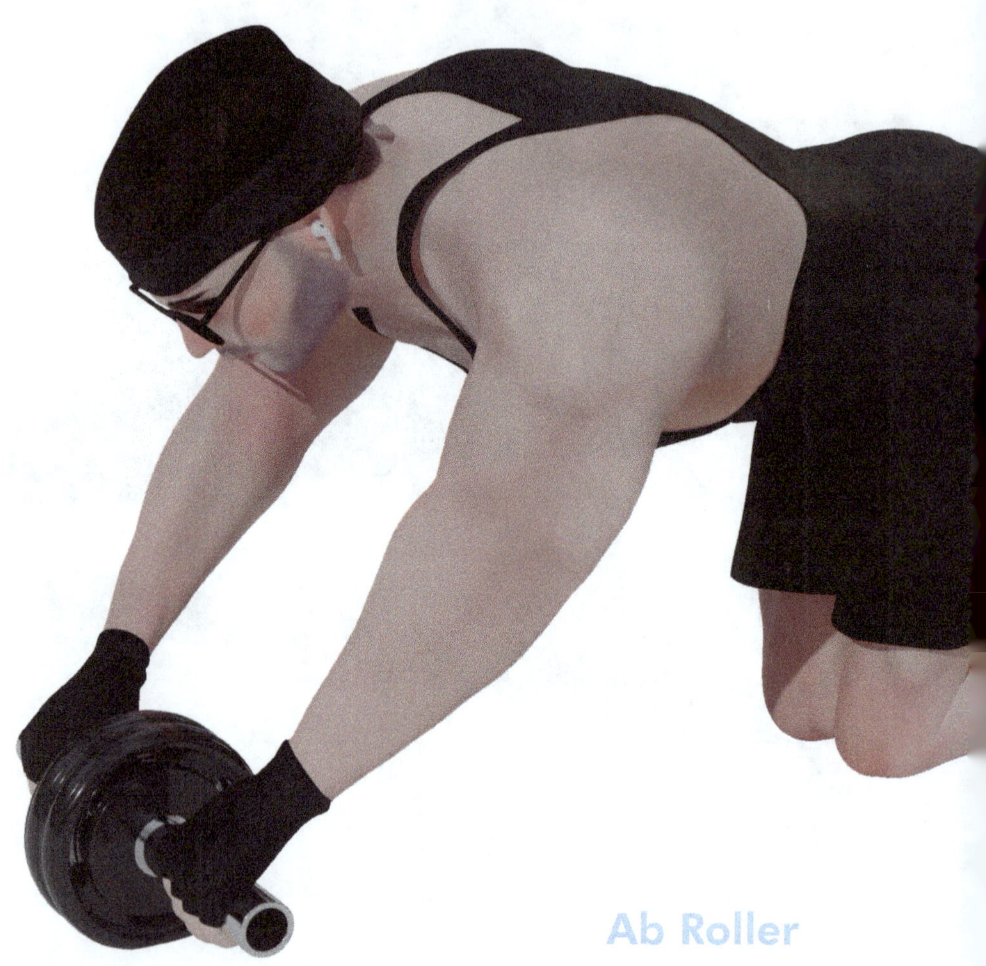

Ab Roller

CORE GROUPING IV

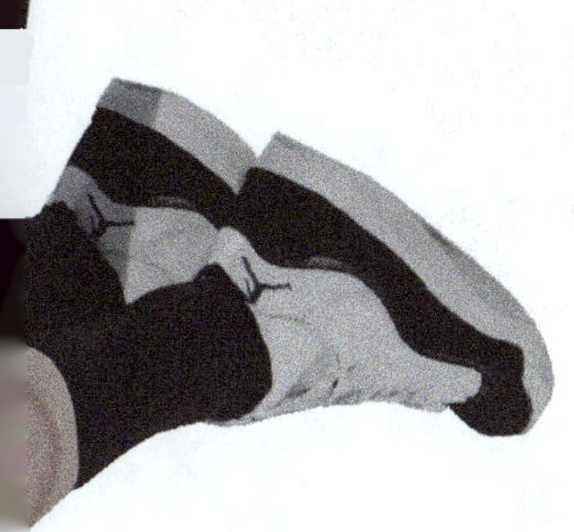

Ab Crunch Machine

Ab Roller

Mountain Climbers

Scissor Kicks

CORE GROUPING V

6"

Pall of Press

TRX Suspended Crunches

Knees to Chest

TRX Suspended Oblique Crunches

Knees to Shoulder Height

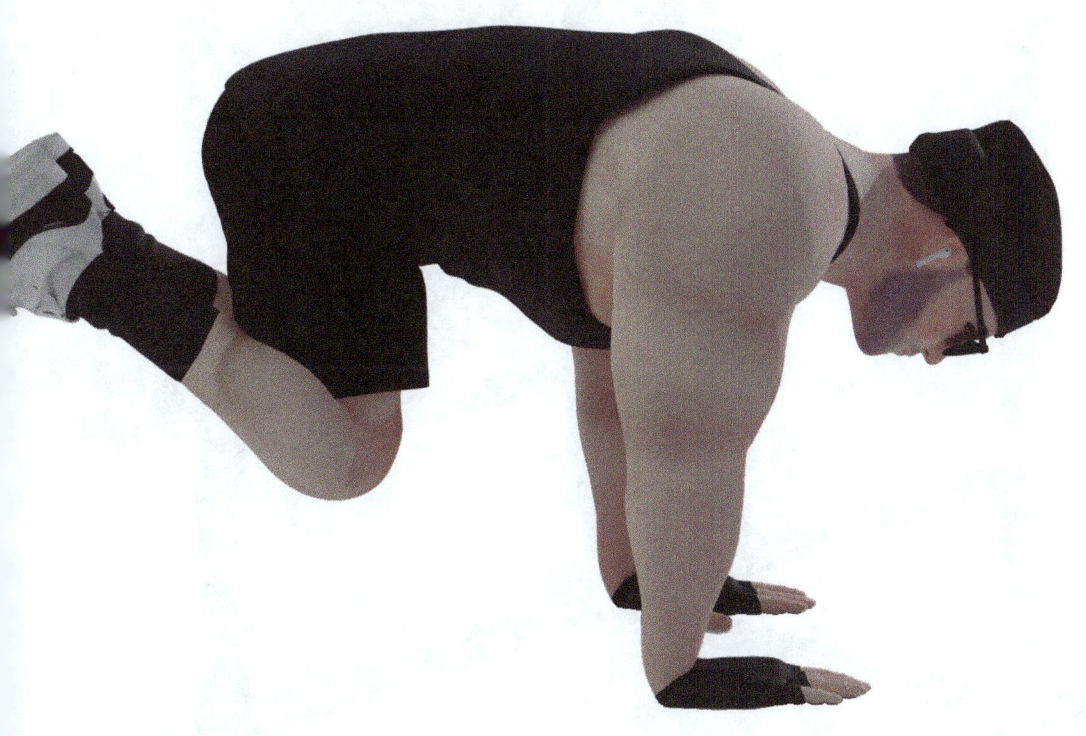

TRX Suspended Crunches

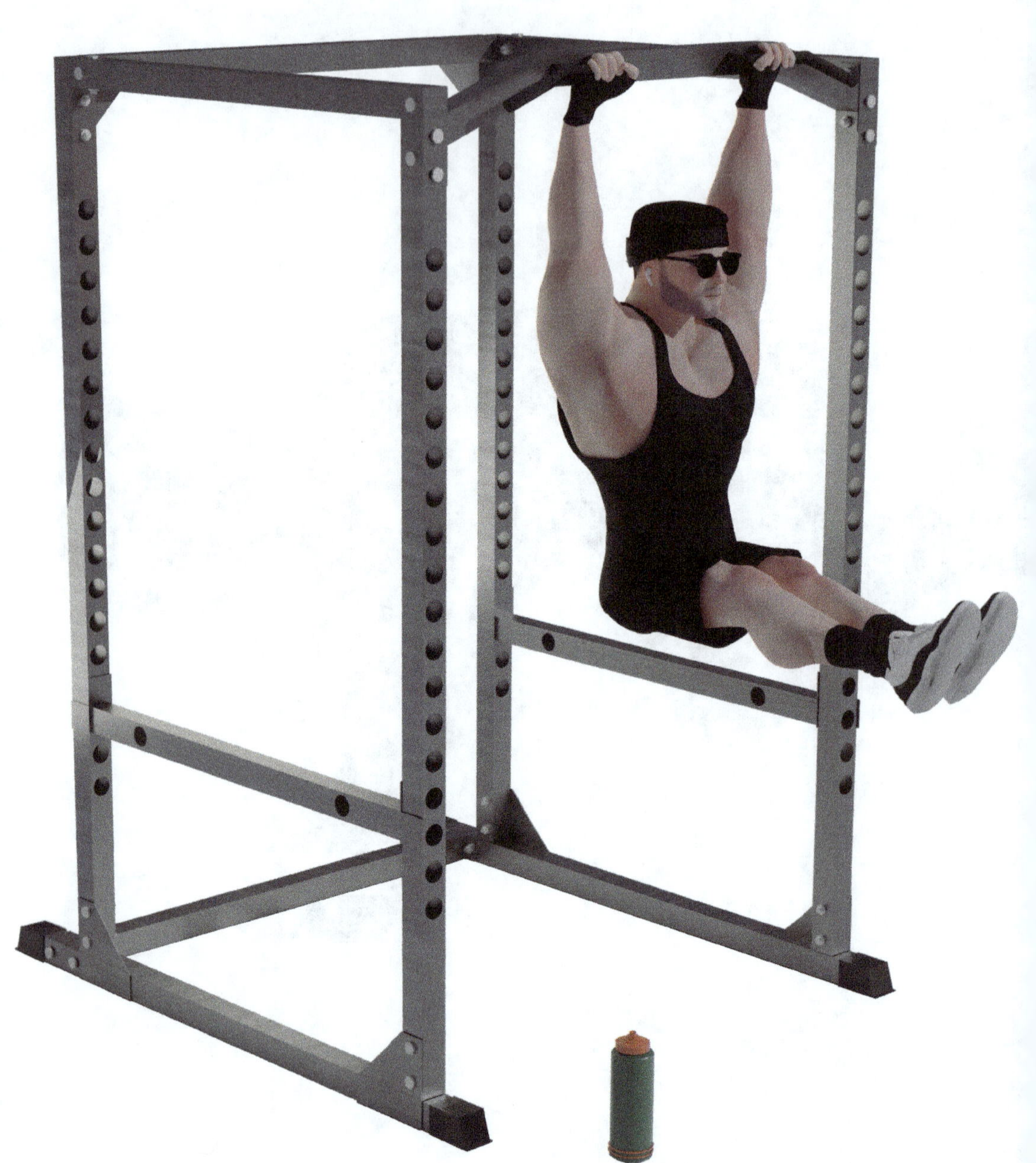

Hanging Windshield Wipers

CORE GROUPING VI

Cross Body Sit-Ups
Back on Floor, Foot on Opposite Bent Knee

Hanging Windshield Wipers

Reverse Cable Wood Chop
1-Knee on Floor (Bottom Inside Hip) to Upper Outside Shoulder

Toe-Touch Crunches
Lower Back Stays Flat on Ground

NO-NOS

Do not repeat the same Grouping Type until you have gone through all the different Groupings.

So if on Tuesday, you picked Core Grouping I and II, do not choose these 2 Groupings until you have cycled through Core Grouping III, IV, V and VI.

PURCHASE A PULL-UP BAR

Try to do 3 sets of 10 pull-ups every single morning and night as an extra exercise. You will soon see the benefits of this add-on!

REST DAY

Having a day off is as important as the exercise days. The relaxation you experience gives you the stamina to be dedicated throughout the workout cycle. It's a vital space to focus on yourself and slow down. Whatever you do with this day, make it count. Enjoy it and don't let it demotivate you. Sometimes when we change our daily routine, it's easy to get lazy. Try and see this rest day as part of the fitness program. This way you will be eager to restart working out the next day! If you start feeling demotivated, be kind to yourself. It's not about being perfect, it's about making progress, slowly but surely.

FOOD IS KEY

One of the most valuable lessons I learned during my ten-year journey was that no matter how diligent I was about sticking to my 5-day workout cycle, my results would not be achieved unless my eating habits changed. This way I could help my body achieve its goal.

It might be handy to monitor your food and drinks by having a food journal so you can keep track of what you are eating and when. If you have any health conditions, make sure you speak to your doctor before cutting anything out.

Some books are certainly much more detailed but I found that sticking to the following eating regiment was the only way for me to get the results I wanted.

Here is an example of a possible daily diet. The main idea is to stay away from heavy carbs like white carbs (white bread, rice or pasta), not to eat after 9pm and to avoid dairy and alcohol. My daily food intake is based on an intermittent fasting routine. It means I only eat between 11am and 9pm. This way of eating might not work for everyone but it helped me.

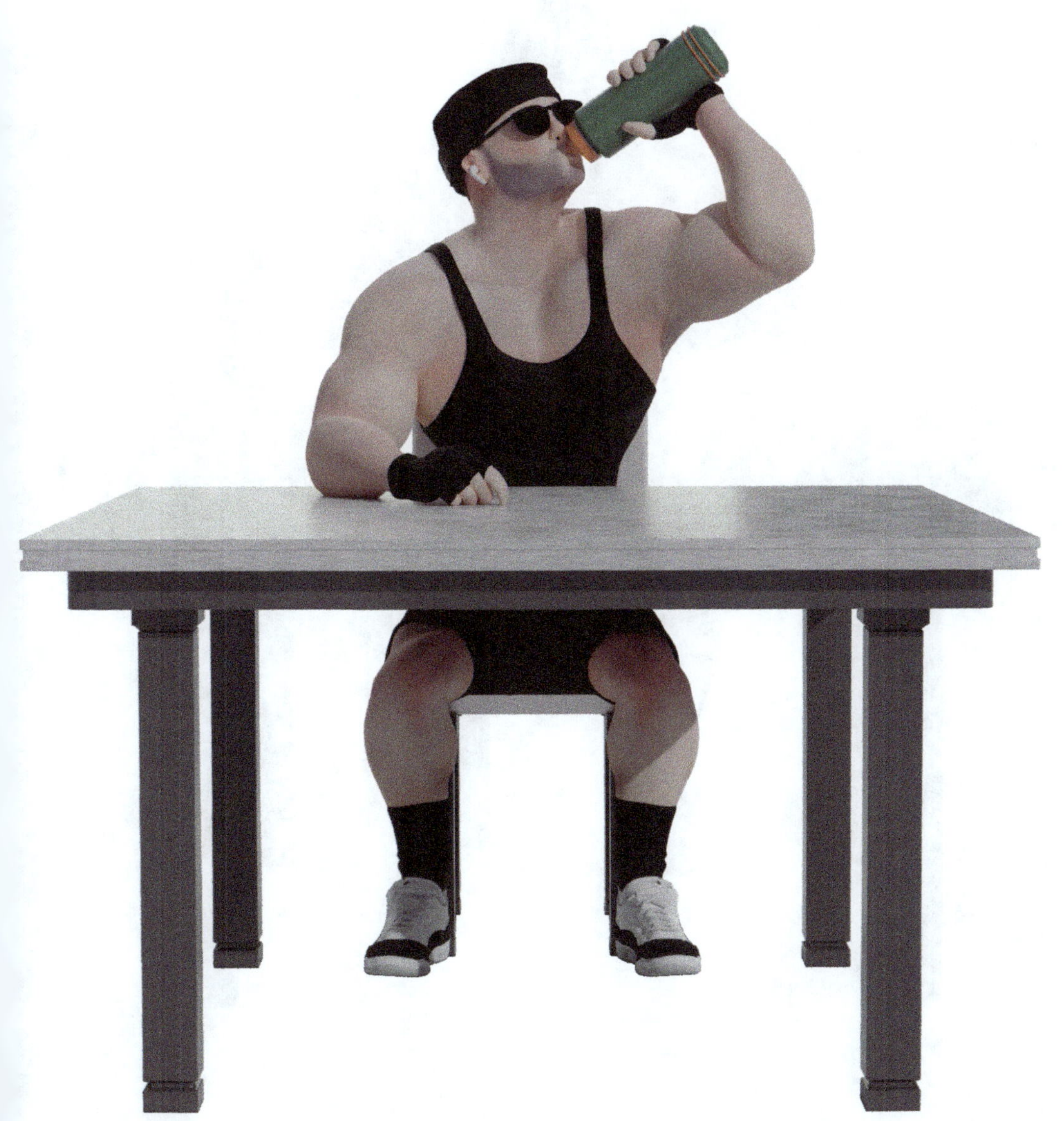

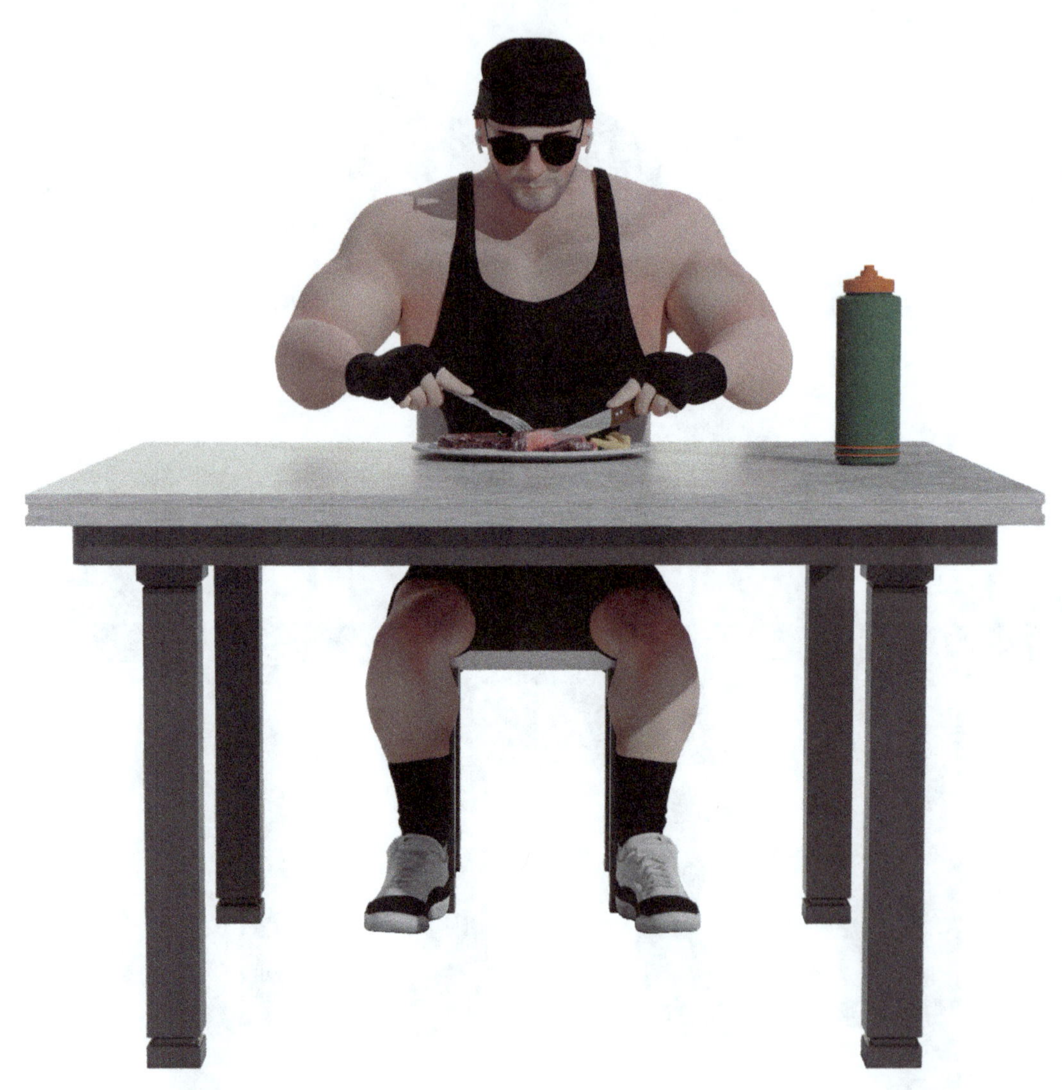

BREAKFAST
Water
Coffee (black preferably)/Tea

Eggs
Protein Bar
Fruit

LUNCH/DINNER
Salad
Chicken/Steak/Fish
Peanut Butter & Jelly

*Sides can include any assortment
of vegetables*

If you need to have carbs, make sure they are complex so
brown rice, brown pasta, but avoid bread and limit your
amount per meal. Drink plenty of water throughout the
day and avoid energy drinks. They sometimes have very
high amounts of caffeine.

Maximize all of the minutes, hours and seconds that you dedicate to this fitness routine. Once you repeat the cycle a few times, you will start seeing results. If it takes longer, don't get discouraged. Make sure you always stretch and give yourself time to meditate and relax your mind. If you're like me, that'll entail some headphones plugged in your ears, feeling the breeze as it passes by.

Remember why you are putting all these efforts in and be kind to your body. If today was not as good as yesterday, show compassion. Nothing is ever perfect but putting a real and honest effort in will bring you closer to achieving the body you want—your perfect body, not the one you see in the media. Work hard, push yourself and don't forget it's the overall progress line that counts!

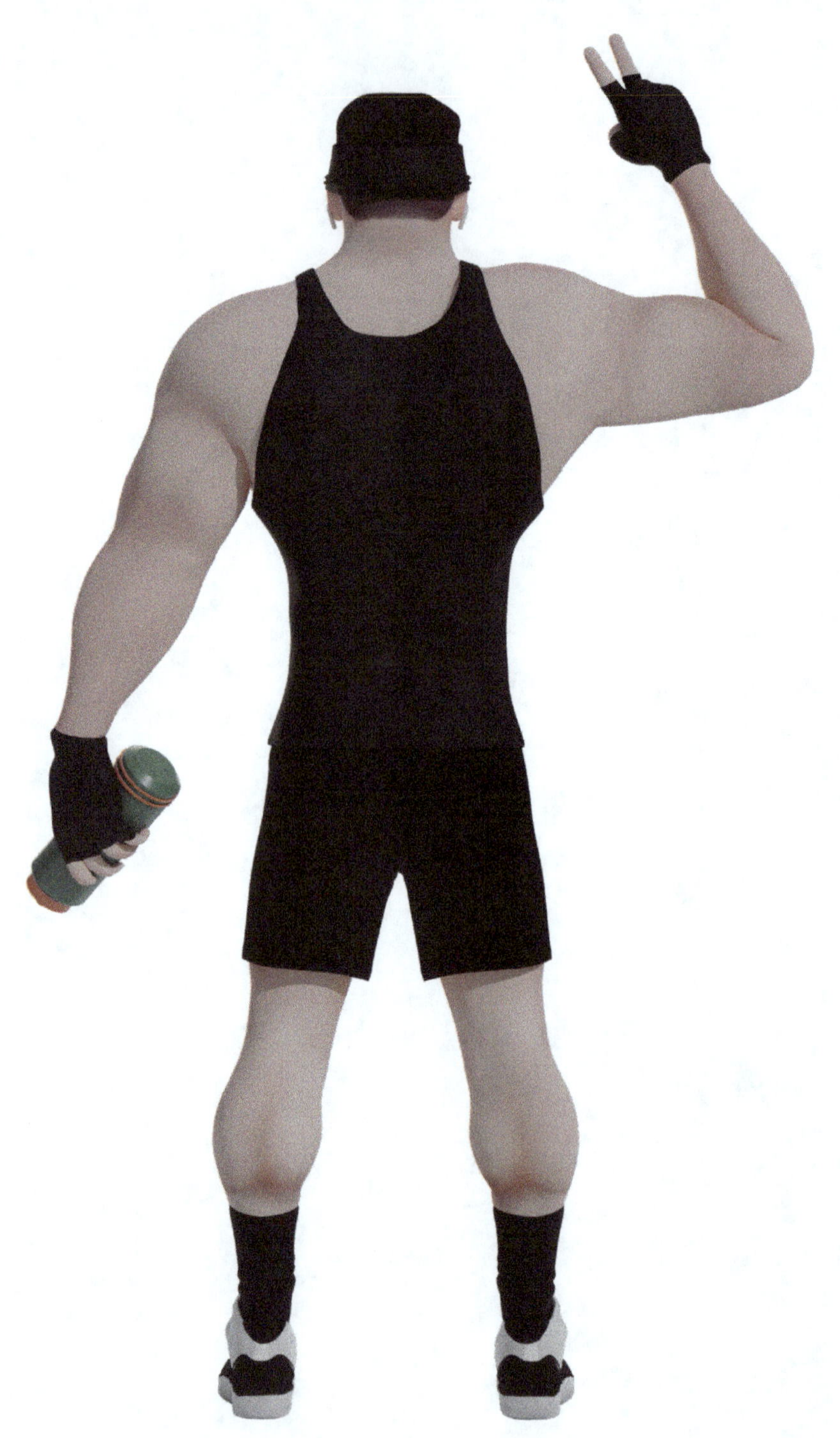

With all my love,

JRusChocolateChipMusic@gmail.com

ChocolateChipMusic.com